Practical Epidemiology

T.

MEDICINE IN THE TROPICS SERIES

Already published

Tropical Venereology, Second edition
O. P. Arya, A. O. Osoba and F. J. Bennett

Leprosy, Third edition
Antony Bryceson and Roy E. Pfaltzgraff

Epidemiology and the Community Control of Disease in Warm Climate Countries, Second edition
Derek Robinson

Diagnostic Pathways in Clinical Medicine, Second edition
B. J. Essex

Leprosy
Edited by Robert C. Hastings

Medicine in the Tropics, Second edition
Edited by A. M. Woodruff and S. G. Wright

Practical Epidemiology

D. J. P. Barker BSc PhD MD FRCP FFCM
Director and Professor of Clinical Epidemiology,
Medical Research Council
Environmental Epidemiology Unit,
Southampton University, UK

A. J. Hall MSc PhD MRCP
Epidemiologist,
IARC, Banjul,
The Gambia, West Africa.

FOURTH EDITION

CHURCHILL LIVINGSTONE
EDINBURGH LONDON MELBOURNE AND NEW YORK 1991

CHURCHILL LIVINGSTONE
Medical Division of Longman Group UK Limited

Distributed in the United States of America by Churchill
Livingstone Inc., 1560 Broadway, New York, N.Y. 10036,
and by associated companies, branches and representatives
throughout the world.

First edition 1973
Second edition 1976
Third edition 1982
Fourth edition 1991

ISBN 0-443-03787-6

British Library Cataloguing in Publication Data
Barker, D. J. P. (David James Purslove)
  Epidemiology in medical practice – 4th ed
  1. Man. Diseases. Epidemiology
  I. Title II. Rose, Geoffrey *1926*– III. Series 614.4

Library of Congress Cataloging in Publication Data
Barker, D. J. P. (David James Purslove)
    Practical epidemiology/D. J. P. Barker, A. J. Hall. – 4th ed.
      p. cm. – (Medicine in the tropics series)
    Includes bibliographical references.
    Includes index.
    ISBN 0-443-03787-6
    1. Epidemiology – Technique. I. Hall, A. J. (Andrew James)
  II. Title. III. Series: Medicine in the tropics.
    [DNLM: 1. Epidemiology. WA 105 B255p]
  RA652.4.B37 1991
  614.4′0723–dc20
  DNLM/DLC
  for Library of Congress   90–2015

Printed in Malaysia by Sun U Book Co., Sdn. Bhd.,
Petaling Jaya, Selangor Darul Ehsan.

Preface

This book, first published in 1972, attempts to meet the need for a short practical manual of epidemiology for use in developing countries. The earlier editions owed much to Professor F. J. Bennett, at that time Professor of Preventive Medicine at Makerere University, Uganda. He wrote the chapters on fieldwork techniques and investigation of epidemics and his wide knowledge and experience benefited other parts of the book.

Dr A. J. Hall, who works in West Africa, is co-author of this fourth edition. We have revised the text throughout, paying particular attention to new techniques of data collection and analysis made possible by computers.

Southampton 1991   D. J. P. B.
                                                                    A. J. H.

Contents

1. The purpose and methods of epidemiology

THE PURPOSE

Epidemiology may be defined as the study of the distribution and determinants of disease in human populations. Whereas the basis of clinical research is the observation of individual patients, epidemiology requires observation of communities of people among whom disease occurs. Historically epidemiology arose out of the study of epidemic diseases such as plague, cholera and scurvy, but its scope has now expanded to include all diseases, irrespective of whether their frequency shows epidemic fluctuations.

The purposes for which epidemiological investigations are carried out may be considered under five headings, although a single investigation may in fact serve more than one purpose.

1. Provision of data necessary for planning and evaluating health care
2. Identification of determinants of disease so as to enable prevention
3. Evaluation of methods used to control disease
4. Description of the natural history of disease
5. Classification of disease.

The techniques of epidemiology can also be applied to the study of the *distribution of biological characteristics* such as body weight and blood groups. The purpose of these investigations is to reveal the normal characteristics of populations rather than abnormal ones related to disease.

Planning and evaluating health care

The lack of basic data on the frequency and distribution of different diseases within developing countries makes it difficult to effect a rational allocation of the limited resources available for disease prevention and patient care. Too many hospitals have been built, equipped and staffed without knowledge of the particular disease problems affecting the communities they are intended to serve. Systems of community medical care have been elaborated which are inappropriate to the needs of the people. In all countries there is a continuing need for numerical data on disease distribution to determine priorities for the health services and ensure that the activities of medical staff are in accord with these priorities.

In the same way as a sick person requires diagnosis, treatment and continued observation, so a community requires recognition of its health problems, the operation of appropriate preventive or curative health services and continued observation to ensure that these services are effective. All stages of community medicine depend upon epidemiological information.

A complete description of the health problems of a community will comprise an account not only of the distribution and frequency of different diseases, but also of the community's view of its own problems and its use of existing health services. Epidemiological studies are required to measure several indices of health. A community's *need* for health services is measured by the frequency of disease, and the occurrence of groups, such as primiparous pregnant women, who have a special need for health care. Analysis of the *utilization* of health services, for example the number of clinic attendances, may require study of such factors as the community's preference for government medical services as opposed to traditional healers, or the methods used for excreta disposal, or attitudes to leprosy. The *effectiveness* of health services is measured by the resulting reduction in disability or death.

Definition of the community's health problems does not, of itself, ensure that an appropriate health service comes into action. Adequate funds and staff must be available, and these are especially limited in developing countries. Priority has to be given to one part of the preventive and curative services at the expense of another. Funds may be insufficient to provide adequate facilities for all surgical emergencies as well as a control programme for tuberculosis.

Major decisions about the allocation of funds are usually made by politicians, and are therefore subject to political influence of all kinds. Nevertheless governments in Africa are only able to make reasoned decisions about funds for control of acquired immune deficiency syndrome (AIDS) once epidemiological surveys reveal the extent of the problem, the uneven distribution of the disease, and the predicted frequency in the future.

Funds and personnel may not be available for surveys of disease prevalence on a national scale or for implementation of recommendations on health services arising from these surveys. But even limited epidemiological surveys can be used to practical advantage by making medical activities appropriate to the community's needs. A medical officer who studies the epidemiology of disease in his local community may find that conditions such as heart failure and intestinal obstruction, to which he devotes much of his time in the clinics and hospital, are not those which impose the major burden on the health of the people. He may therefore decide to reallocate his time so that, for example, he spends less time in the operating theatre and more time immunizing children or treating gonorrhoea in clinics away from the hospital. An obstetrician may find that, despite the high standards of obstetric care maintained within his hospital, the number of babies stillborn or dying shortly after birth in the area as a whole is no lower than that in neighbouring areas without access to a hospital. He may decide therefore to apportion fewer nursing staff to the hospital unit and more to teaching birth attendants in the villages.

Identification of the determinants of disease

It is a commonplace to state that the occurrence of a disease is determined by many influences, and that inadequate ventilation in houses and a poor diet are as much 'causes' of tuberculosis as the organism *Mycobacterium tuberculosis*. The main purpose of epidemiological studies of disease causation is to identify those determinants whose manipulation could lead to prevention rather than those such as genetic constitution which, although of great interest, cannot be manipulated at the present time.

Hypotheses about disease causation may arise directly out of a simple epidemiological description of a disease in terms of the kind of people affected by it (e.g. their age, sex, occupation), its geographical distribution, and the variation in its frequency of occurrence at different times. An example of such a hypothesis is the suggestion that the development of Burkitt's lymphoma is related to previous malarial infection. This idea arose from the observation that the geographical distribution of the two diseases was similar. The similarity between the distribution of cancer of the mouth and the practice of chewing tobacco has led to the conclusion that they are causally related. Marked differences in the frequency of oesophageal cancer in neighbouring communities has led to a search for determinants among those factors in which the communities differ, and as a result locally brewed alcoholic drinks are suspected of containing carcinogens.

Although epidemiological studies may give rise to new hypotheses about disease causation, more often they are used to test hypotheses generated from other research methods. In the early years of this century there were two theories explaining the aetiology of pellagra. It was thought to be either dietary in origin, in some way associated with the ingestion of maize, or an infectious disease communicable from one person to another. But observations made in asylums and other institutions in Italy and the USA showed that, whereas pellagra was common among the patients, it did not affect their attendants. This finding was hardly compatible with the theory of an infectious disease but was readily explained by the different diets of the attendants and patients.

Evaluation of methods of disease control

It may seem scarcely necessary to state that any measures taken to control a disease must be accompanied by methods for assessing whether these measures are effective in reducing the frequency of the disease. Just as any programme for eradication of tsetse flies includes regular counts of the number of tsetse flies remaining in the area, so must a national campaign against gonorrhoea be supported by repeated estimates of the numbers of cases in the country. This simple principle is too often ignored in disease control. International agencies, for example, have in the past seemed content to give away large quantities of free milk without verifying that the milk was fulfilling its purpose by reducing childhood malnutrition.

Evaluation of a new control method such as bed nets impregnated with insecticide in the control of malaria, requires more than the demonstration of its effectiveness in reducing disease frequency. It is necessary to measure the cost of its large-scale application in terms of trained personnel, time required, money needed for basic materials and transport, and other factors. The value of one method in relation to others is assessed by relating the cost of its application to its effectiveness. The *cost-effectiveness* of bed nets is being compared with that of other methods such as chemoprophylaxis.

Usually the task of evaluating large-scale control measures will fall to full-time epidemiologists and statisticians working for governments or organizations such as the World Health Organization (WHO). But health education is one example of a disease control method which has been the subject of numerous interesting experiments carried out by doctors working in the clinical services. For instance, mothers attending antenatal clinics have been given courses of instruction on infant feeding in an attempt to prevent kwashiorkor. The effectiveness of this instruction may be evaluated by measurement of a decline in kwashiorkor, and of a change in the knowledge, attitudes and behaviour which the instruction is intended to influence. But too often the arguments which support one method of health education as being more effective than another are based on opinion and conjecture, rather than measurements of change in disease frequency or in some relevant aspect of behaviour following use of the method.

Observation of the natural history of disease

It is seldom that a doctor is able to follow the course of a chronic disease from its inception to its termination. Doctors tend to see only those more seriously affected by a disease, and their relationship with one patient usually does not extend over a prolonged period. There is much to be learnt about the natural history of even such intensively studied diseases as peptic ulcer and diabetes.

Knowledge of disease natural history is essential since without it a doctor cannot make a *prognosis* of the likely outcome of a patient's illness. This prognosis is the basis for rational decisions about therapy. Studies of the natural history of chronic disease require repeated observations made over many years in communities where the disease occurs. Long-term studies of this kind are time-consuming and expensive. However, they have been used to resolve problems such as the prognosis of tropical sprue, and to explore the interaction between infectious disease and protein–calorie malnutrition. They are the only method of determining whether the pathogenicity of the two human immuno-deficiency viruses (HIV) that cause AIDS, that is, HIV_1 and HIV_2, is different.

Classification of disease

The epidemiological characteristics of a disease are an integral part of its basic description, by means of which it is defined and recognized. For example, kuru (a fatal disease due to degeneration of the central nervous system, particularly the cerebellum) was defined as a clinical entity partly by its restriction to the Fore people in the Eastern Highlands of New Guinea. When one considers the many undiagnosed tropical disorders vaguely attributed to viruses, or the difficulties in classifying tropical skin diseases, there seems little doubt that study of the epidemiological characteristics of patients with apparently similar clinical presentations will lead to the recognition of many new tropical disease entities.

THE METHODS OF EPIDEMIOLOGY

The intention in carrying out an epidemiological investigation of a disease may be either to *describe* its pattern of occurrence in a population or to *analyse* the influences which determine that one person is affected while another is not. Although a single study can be designed to provide both descriptive and analytic data, in practice the design of a study is mainly determined by the need to obtain data of one or other kinds.

Descriptive studies

Descriptive studies are carried out in order to determine the frequency of a disease, the kind of people suffering from it, and where and when it occurs. Information about patients is analysed to show the distribution of attributes or variables such as their sex and age, and the time and place where they developed the disease. An *attribute* is a quality or characteristic of a person — e.g. sex, whereas a *variable* is a quantity which may vary in value — e.g. age.

Such studies are often based upon hospital records, and in these circumstances patients can be characterized only in terms of simple variables or attributes which are recorded in case notes, i.e. age, sex, marital status, occupation and place of residence. Using hospital records the geographical distribution of a disease, and any variations in its occurrence at different times of the year, can be deduced only in so far as they are reflected in the home addresses given by the patients and the dates when they were admitted to hospital. If, however, a descriptive study comprises interview and examination of the patients by the investigator, then more specific information can be obtained. For example, patients can be tabulated according to the month of the year when their first symptom or sign appeared rather than the month when they came to the hospital — a refinement which would make little difference in a study of acute diseases such as meningococcal meningitis, but would lead to a more accurate description of any seasonal variation in a chronic disease such as trachoma.

Descriptive studies seek to characterize people affected by a disease, and it is therefore necessary to relate observations made on the patients to similar observations made on the general population. For example, there may be twice as many children as adults suffering from a disease either because the disease has a predilection for children, or because there are twice as many children as adults in the population as a whole. It is a particular difficulty of epidemiology in developing countries that basic census data on the numbers, characteristics and distribution of peoples are often not available.

A descriptive study will usually comprise observations made at one point in time, so-called *cross-sectional studies*. However there is an increasing emphasis on the value of *longitudinal studies* in which observations are repeated in the same community over a prolonged period. A number of longitudinal studies have been carried out in which children have been regularly observed over a period of many years and the patterns of development and sickness among them described.

Descriptive studies yield information which is of immediate relevance to the planning of medical services, and to disease classification and natural history. In aetiological enquiries they sometimes lead immediately to a specific hypothesis, and the suspected relationship between Burkitt's tumour and malaria is an example of this. More frequently they indicate problems that demand further study. For instance, there are marked geographical variations in the frequency of certain cancers. Colonic cancer is rare in Japan but common in North America, and in the Japanese communities who have emigrated there. These variations suggest that a search for environmental determinants of the cancer may be rewarding.

In infectious and parasitic diseases descriptive epidemiological studies are an essential part of the information needed for understanding of the inter-relationship between the environment, the disease agent and the human host. In the search for the species of *Phlebotomus* acting as vector of kala-azar in East Africa the seasonal pattern of the disease was correlated with the seasonal habits of possible vectors. When potential vector breeding sites, such as termite mounds, were considered the age and sex distribution of the patients was related to the relative frequency with which men and women, adults and children, came into the proximity of these sites.

Analytic studies

Analytic studies are carried out to test hypotheses about the influences which determine that one person is affected by a disease while another is not. They are designed to show whether particular events (such as consumption of certain foods), or states (such as living in overcrowded houses), act as 'causes' whose 'effect' is the resulting disease. Thorough discussion of the concepts of cause and effect is a matter for philosophers; but it is unnecessary to digress into this issue in order to solve the practical problems of an epidemiological study.

There are two basic kinds of epidemiological observation made on groups of people which suggest that a particular event or state is a determinant of a particular disorder. As an example one may consider evidence which would suggest that a diet composed largely of maize is a determinant of pellagra.

1. *Comparison of people with the disorder and normal people, showing that the determinant occurs more frequently among those with the disorder than those without it.* Among a group of people with pellagra there will be a greater proportion of individuals eating a maize diet than there will be among a comparable group of people not affected by the disease.

2. *Comparison of people exposed to the determinant and those not exposed, showing that a greater proportion of people develop the disease among the exposed group than among the non-exposed.* If two populations are compared, in one of which (population A) the people live on a maize diet while in the other (population B) the people live on meat and vegetables, or some other diet, then there will be a greater proportion of people with the disorder in population A than in population B.

Either of these two types of observation will suggest that maize diets and pellagra are *associated*, i.e. not independent of one another, but this is not proof that a maize diet actually determines the occurrence of pellagra in an individual. Maize diets and pellagra are both characteristics of the way of life of people in certain impoverished rural communities. It could be suggested that pellagra is associated with maize diets only in the same way as it is associated with many other characteristics of these communities, such as poor sanitation or lack of shoes. Clearly two states, or events, can be associated without one being a cause of the other. The proof that maize diets are a determinant of pellagra comes from additional sources of evidence, such as knowledge of nicotinic acid metabolism and observation of the prevention of pellagra by alterations in the diet. An analytic epidemiological study is usually completed when a suspected determinant and a disorder are shown to be associated. Further investigation of this association will depend upon work in other branches of research or upon further epidemiological studies designed to answer specific questions about the relationship between the determinant and the disorder. The strongest epidemiological evidence for causation comes from a randomized trial of prevention in which only one suspected cause is changed (Ch. 10).

*Case-control and cohort studies

In the preceding section it has been stated that there are two basic kinds of epidemiological observation which can suggest that a particular event or state is associated with and may be a determinant of a disorder. The first type of observation depends upon comparison between people with the disorder and those without, while the second type depends upon comparison between people exposed to the suspected determinant and those not exposed. Corresponding with these two kinds of observation there are two methods used for analytic epidemiological studies. In *case-control studies* the starting point is the identification of a group of people who have the disease. *Cohort studies* begin with identification of a group of people who are exposed to the suspected determinant. A *cohort* is defined as a group of people sharing a common experience.

During the early investigations into the aetiology of pellagra a comparison was made between the diet of a group of patients suffering from pellagra, who came from a poor rural area of the USA, and the diet of a group of people from a nearby city slum who did not have pellagra. It was shown that among the pellagra patients there was a higher proportion living on an unvaried, mainly maize diet, than among the slum-dwellers. This is an example of a case-control study involving comparison of a group of patients with a group of controls (the slum-dwellers).

A cohort study on the same problem comprised observation of two groups of people in a state sanatorium. The residents of the sanatorium had a mainly cereal diet, while their attendants had a diet with more meat and vegetables and less cereal. The two groups were observed for a number of years, during which time approximately 10% of the residents developed pellagra while none of their attendants did so.

The two types of study give answers to two different questions. To illustrate this, suppose that an investigation is required to determine whether delivery by obstetric forceps, and the accompanying trauma to the infant's head, can result in brain damage that is manifested as childhood epilepsy. A case-control study would comprise comparison of the obstetric histories of a group of epileptic children with the histories of a control group of non-epileptic children. If the proportion of epileptic children with a history of forceps delivery exceeds the proportion of control children, this suggests that forceps delivery may be a cause of epilepsy. From these two proportions the relative contribution of forceps delivery to the total frequency of epilepsy can be estimated. This is a guide to its importance as a public health problem.

A cohort study of the same problem would compare a group of children delivered by forceps with a group of children delivered normally. If it is found that the proportion a of forceps-delivered children who developed epilepsy exceeds the proportion b of normally delivered children then this suggests that forceps delivery is associated with and may be a determinant of epilepsy. But forceps delivery does not invariably lead to epilepsy, which occurs in only a proportion of children delivered in this way. The difference in the proportion $(a - b)$ represents the statistical risk of epilepsy developing as a consequence of forceps delivery. This is known as the *attributable risk* and is a guide to the management of individual patients.

The magnitude of the effect, or strength, of a suspected cause can conveniently be expressed as a/b, which is known as the *relative risk*. Whereas in a cohort study this can be calculated directly, in a case-control study it can only be estimated indirectly.

Both types of study may be used to show whether a disease and a suspected determinant are associated, and therefore perhaps causally related. But analysis of this association by a case-control study will show *the proportion of cases of the disease which may be caused by the determinant*. Analysis by a cohort study will show *the proportion of people in whom exposure to the determinant results in development of the disease*.

In practice one must choose whether to use the case-control or cohort method during an investigation, and in part this choice will be determined by what is feasible. Case-control studies can often be carried out quickly and cheaply, since the identification of a group of people suffering from a disease may be easily effected through hospitals or clinics. On the other hand, cohort studies begin with the identification of people who are not affected by a disorder at the time of their selection and who regard themselves as healthy. Subsequent observations are made on these people over a period of time, often over years. If exposure to the determinant is only rarely followed by the development of the disease it will be necessary to observe a large number of people. For these reasons many cohort studies are expensive and can only be undertaken by people with a full-time commitment to the project. However, if the disorder is common and follows exposure to the determinant by only a few weeks or months it may be possible to execute a cohort study inexpensively and swiftly. In general, case-control studies are used for exploratory investigations of disease determinants and cohort studies are reserved for examination of particular suspected causes.

Experimental studies

In many branches of science progress depends upon an orderly sequence of formulation of hypotheses followed by design and execution of experiments to test the hypotheses. Epidemiologists study human populations and therefore are generally unable to carry out experiments. They depend upon observation of changes and events whose occurrence is outside their control. However, experiments are sometimes feasible and Chapter 10 describes the methods used in experimental trials of preventive measures such as vaccines.

Definition of objectives

In the following chapters an account will be given of the methods by which epidemiological studies are carried out. Many of the difficulties encountered in these studies can be avoided if the investigator clearly defines the objectives at the outset. Is it a purely descriptive study? If it is an analytic study what precisely are the questions that the study seeks to answer? There must be few epidemiologists or medical statisticians who, having been asked to assist with the analysis of a completed study, have not found on occasion that even in this final stage of an investigation the investigator can only state in general terms the original purpose for making the study.

ADMINISTRATION OF AN EPIDEMIOLOGICAL INVESTIGATION

Although each epidemiological investigation has its particular requirements the administrative steps common to many investigations may be categorized under four phases; planning, organization, execution, evaluation and feedback.

Planning   *Pilot Survey.*

1. Define objectives and type of study to be carried out
2. Determine how much money and how many staff are available
3. Look up reports of previous studies and consult people with experience in the particular field
4. Complete national or local formalities necessary to obtain permission for the survey (Ch. 7)
5. Make a preliminary appraisal of the area to obtain demographic, social and cultural data (Ch. 7)
6. Define the observations to be made and choose standardized techniques for making them (Chs 2 and 5)
7. Choose a study population and a method of sampling it (Ch. 3)
8. Choose a method of selecting controls, if necessary (Ch. 4)
9. Decide the timing of the survey (Ch. 7)

Organization

1. Obtain community collaboration (Ch. 7)
2. Select personnel and train them (Chs 2 and 7)
3. Arrange the necessary laboratory facilities (Ch. 7)
4. Work out 'line of flow' (Ch. 7), and design and print records (Ch. 6)
5. Obtain special equipment (with spares), drugs, other medical supplies, etc. List them
6. Organize transport and accommodation of survey staff (Ch. 7)
7. Try out survey procedures to assess their acceptability to local population, and to test techniques (Ch. 2)

Execution

1. Supervise staff and ensure the continuing accuracy of observation and recording (Ch. 7)
2. Ensure the continuing co-operation of the population (Ch. 7)

Evaluation and feedback

1. Analyse data during the course of the investigation and consequently modify techniques, re-allocate personnel, alter time tables, etc. (Chs 7 and 8)
2. Make a final analysis of data and report conclusions to: scientific journals; ministries and other interested bodies; the survey staff and local health workers; the survey population and its leaders (Ch. 8).

2. Making observations and counting diseases

MAKING OBSERVATIONS

As with all scientific observations the results of an epidemiological study must be amenable to evaluation by persons other than the investigator. It is therefore necessary for the investigator to define the precision with which observations are made. Consider, for example, the findings of a morbidity survey which showed that out of 500 children examined 50 had heart murmurs. One cannot deduce that 10% of the children had a cardiovascular abnormality, for the significance of the observations depends entirely on the circumstances under which they were made. A cardiologist will probably record more murmurs than a general duties medical officer. More murmurs can be heard when examination is carried out in a quiet clinic room than will be heard during a village survey. Many normal children have cardiac murmurs and criteria must be laid down to define what murmurs are regarded as pathological. Clearly, observations on the frequency of heart murmurs are of no value unless they are _standardized_, that is carried out in such a way that they can be directly compared with other observations made by other observers.

Standardized methods of observation and recording are essential in epidemiology, and before commencing any study it is necessary to:

1. decide what observations to make;
2. choose a suitable technique;
3. train personnel to use the technique;
4. test the technique.

The problems of measuring body weight are simple in comparison with those of assessing nutritional status. But even for recording weight a standardized technique must be worked out by reference to the four headings given above. Accordingly it is necessary to:

1. decide whether to weigh all the people in the survey, or only particular subgroups;
2. choose scales that are sufficiently accurate and robust, and decide whether to weigh the people fully or partially clothed;
3. ensure that whoever weighs the people can read the scale to the correct number of decimals, can record weight accurately, knows which people to weigh and can periodically check the scales against known standards;
4. test the procedure in the field before starting the survey, and ensure that the procedure is carried out correctly thereafter.

Deciding what observations to make

When consulted by a patient with a chronic cough a doctor must carry out every clinical and laboratory test necessary to exclude pulmonary tuberculosis (TB). When confronted by a community in which an unknown proportion of people have pulmonary TB the doctor must carry out the minimum number of tests necessary to measure the occurrence of the disease with a sufficient degree of accuracy. In order to measure the prevalence of TB in a country, as a preliminary to a programme of disease control, it is unnecessary to identify every case of the disease among the people examined. Instead of exposing every individual to full clinical examination, Mantoux test, sputum examination and chest X-ray, it is often sufficient to use sputum examination alone. The epidemiologist can accept that a proportion of people with a disease will be unrecognized during the survey because, unlike the clinician, he is not required to take immediate action about the health of every individual whom he examines. Instead of the detailed examination of patients appropriate to the clinic or hospital, epidemiologists practise a limited examination whose essential requirement is feasibility for use on large numbers of people, often in places far from the aids and conveniences of a hospital. The epidemiologist accepts that his techniques of observation will not identify all cases of a disease, but at the same time he is careful to specify the limits of the errors which may be made and to ensure that the number of undiagnosed cases is not so great as to bias or distort his findings grossly.

If a group of 100 people was examined to determine the prevalence of active pulmonary TB the following results might be obtained using as alternative methods tuberculin testing, chest X-rays, and sputum examination.

Total number of people in group	100
Number tuberculin-positive	50
Number with chest X-rays showing evidence of TB	6
Number with tubercle bacilli in sputum	1

Almost all people with active pulmonary TB will be tuberculin-positive, but the majority of people who are tuberculin-positive do not have active disease. Tuberculin testing is therefore said to be a *sensitive* test for active pulmonary TB but not a *specific* one. Chest X-ray is less sensitive than tuberculin testing, since a proportion of patients with active disease do not have radiological changes, but is more specific in that the proportion of patients with active disease among those with positive X-rays is higher than among those with positive tuberculin reactions. Nevertheless, on average four out of six persons who have X-ray changes are found to have inactive lesions or some lung disease other than TB. Sputum microscopy and culture is the most specific method but the least sensitive, since tubercle bacilli are found in the sputum of only 70% of patients with active pulmonary TB.

The balance between the sensitivity and specificity required in a particular test depends upon the purpose of the particular survey. Although sputum examination is not the most sensitive test for TB it is nevertheless valuable for public health work since it identifies patients who are coughing out bacilli and therefore spreading the disease. In general, methods of low specificity are avoided since the incorrect inclusion of large numbers of persons with conditions other than the one being investigated renders analysis of the distribution of the disorder liable to error. But an inexpensive non-specific test such as the Venereal Disease Research Laboratories (VDRL) test for syphilis may be useful in screening out those upon whom a more expensive but more specific test, such as the *Treponema pallidum* immobilization test, is required. This removes the necessity of performing an expensive test on the entire survey population.

Consider 100 patients at a clinic who are suspected of having active pulmonary TB (Table 2.1). A technician first examines a single sputum smear from each and finds that 30 contain acid-fast bacilli. Subsequent culture shows that 35 of the sputa contain tubercle bacilli, of which 25 were positive on microscopy. Figures of this kind can be used to quantitate sensitivity and specificity. In this example one would assume that a positive sputum culture is the absolute index of active infectious pulmonary TB and calibrate sputum microscopy against this standard.

Table 2.1 Sputum findings on 100 patients suspected of having TB

	Culture positive	Culture negative	Total
Microscopy positive	25	5	30
Microscopy negative	10	60	70
Total	35	65	100

The sensitivity of microscopy can be expressed as $100 \times 25/(25 + 10) = 71\%$. This expression relates the number of cases correctly identified by microscopy to the total number of cases. The specificity is expressed as $100 \times 60/(5 + 60) = 92\%$. This relates the number of normal people correctly identified by microscopy to the total number of normal people.

Simple calculations of this kind may be used to determine whether clinical diagnosis is sufficient for the recognition of a disease in an epidemiological study, or whether additional tests, such as biopsy, are required. A clinician would find it unacceptable to depend upon clinical diagnosis alone if he thereby failed to recognize a proportion of patients with a disease. But the epidemiologist can accept this, for his concern is not with the diagnosis of individuals but with the application of simple standardized techniques of observation to populations so as to enable description of the distributions of disorders or characteristics and comparison of these distributions in different populations. In epidemiological studies it is often unnecessary to make measurements with the same precision as that required for clinical work, but it is essential that the degree of imprecision can be at least approximately specified.

Results of the kind shown in Table 2.1 are represented algebraically in Table 2.2. Two indices which may be derived in addition

Table 2.2 Results of sputum examination for acid-fast bacilli

	Culture positive	Culture negative
Microscopy positive	Culture positives correctly identified (a)	False positives (b)
Microscopy negative	False negatives (c)	Culture negatives correctly identified (d)

to sensitivity and specificity are the *predictive value* of a positive test and the predictive value of a negative test. The predictive value of a positive test is calculated as $100 \times a/(a + b)$ and expresses the percentage of patients with positive tests, e.g. sputum microscopy, who have the disease. Conversely the predictive value of a negative test is calculated as $100 \times d/(c + d)$ and expresses the percentage of persons with negative tests who do not have the disease.

As an alternative to predictive values the proportion of *false positives* and *false negatives* may be calculated. Whereas the predictive value of a positive test is calculated from $a/(a + b)$, the proportion of false positives is $b/(a + b)$. Likewise the proportion of false negatives is $c/(c + d)$.

Table 2.3 Glycosuria as a test for diabetes

| | Blood sugar level | | Total |
	Diabetic	Non-diabetic	
Glycosuria present	15	5	20
Glycosuria absent	35	95	130
Total	50	100	150

Table 2.3 shows a study of the use of glycosuria as a screening test for diabetes. Measurement of the blood sugar was used as the *reference test* for diabetes, i.e. the test taken as the absolute index of the disease. One-third of the individuals tested were diabetic. The sensitivity of glycosuria as a screening test was $15/50 = 30\%$ and the specificity $95/100 = 95\%$. The predictive value of glycosuria was $15/20 = 75\%$.

Table 2.4 Glycosuria as a test for diabetes

| | Blood sugar level | | Total |
	Diabetic	Non-diabetic	
Glycosuria present	15	35	50
Glycosuria absent	35	665	700
Total	50	700	750

If, instead of 50 diabetics and 100 non-diabetics, the individuals in the study had comprised 50 diabetics and 700 non-diabetics the results would have been those shown in Table 2.4. Here the sensitivity and specificity are seen to be the same as in Table 2.3, but the predictive value of glycosuria has fallen sharply from 75% to $15/50 = 30\%$.

This simplified example demonstrates how predictive values (and proportions of false positives and negatives) are dependent on the frequency of disease in the group being studied whereas, theoretically at least, sensitivity and specificity remain constant irrespective of the frequency. This conclusion is of practical importance since new diagnostic and screening tests are commonly tried out on groups of hospital patients among whom the frequency of the disease being studied is high. The values of the sensitivity and specificity obtained in such preliminary trials may be used in the design of epidemiological studies on the general population, where disease frequency is usually much lower. The predictive values and proportions of false positives and negatives may not be used in this way.

Although theoretically a test has a fixed sensitivity and specificity, in practice some variation in the values may be observed. The form of a disease seen in hospital patients may differ in extent, severity and other manifestations from the form seen in people still living in the community. Therefore the performance of a test may differ in the hospital and in the community because it is used to detect different types of patient. Before using clinical tests in epidemiological studies it is wise to anticipate such an alteration in performance.

Choosing a suitable technique

The most important consideration when choosing a technique is to ensure that it is standardized. Only in this way can the results obtained in one survey be compared with those obtained in others. If, for example, during a nutrition survey measurements of subcutaneous fat are not made with standard skinfold calipers at one of the standard sites then the measurements will not be comparable to the norms recorded in other populations, and will be of little value in assessing the nutritional status of the community. With biochemical and haematological measurements small differences in technique can result in marked differences in the distribution of series of results from a population. An epidemiologist is incautious if he spends long hours in the field taking blood samples without first verifying that the results of the analysis will be comparable to those of other surveys.

For many diseases there are now standard techniques which can be used to elicit symptoms or signs in a prescribed form and to take standardized measurements.

When it is necessary for an investigator to develop a new technique then this must have the following characteristics:

1. It must be valid, that is it must measure what it is intended to measure. A routine clinical examination to detect nutritional disorders, for example, must be constructed so that it detects as many people as possible who have the disorders while generally excluding those who are normal or have other conditions. *Validity* is therefore compounded of sensitivity and specificity, discussed above.

2. Use of the technique should be practical in the particular circumstances of the survey, i.e. in villages, clinics, mobile units etc.; and it should be sufficiently inexpensive to enable its use on large numbers of people.

3. It should be sufficiently precise for the purpose for which it is intended. Measurement of haemoglobin will give an indication of the prevalence of anaemia in the population, but a complete inquiry may require, in addition, thin and thick blood films and a microhaematocrit.

4. The conditions under which it should be used must be specified. For example, correct lighting is required for tests of visual acuity, and in certain areas the diagnosis of *Wuchereria bancrofti* requires blood samples taken around midnight.

Training the personnel to use the technique

In field studies many of the tasks of organizing records, interviewing, and making simple observations can be carried out by paramedical assistants or with the help of unskilled but intelligent assistance from local administrators, senior secondary schoolchildren, or other groups. Every person assisting in a survey will require some preliminary training. An important part of this will be detailed instruction to ensure that the observations made are not subject to excessive *observer variation*. Observations made by laypeople can be used as a screening test. In surveys of poliomyelitis, for example, headteachers were asked to list children in their school who had a limp. All these children, and a sample of those not listed, were then examined by a doctor to determine if the limp was caused by poliomyelitis.

There are two kinds of observer variation or error. *Between-*

observer variation arises if one observer examines a blood-film and diagnoses malaria, while a second observer examines the same film and finds it normal. *Within-observer variation* arises if a single observer performs two consecutive measurements of arm circumference in the same patient and obtains two different results.

Observer variation may arise during the use of a questionnaire. Two interviewers asking questions about the source of a family's domestic water supply may get differing responses. To an interviewer who is brusque and hurried the family may say that they use the nearby well. A more sympathetic and patient interviewer may elicit the information that, although the well is the main source of supply, during the rains the family uses a seasonal swamp which is nearer to their home than the well, and moreover the older members of the family often go to the river to bathe rather than carry water from the well back to their home. This differing response to two interviewers would give between-observer variation. The same question would be subject to within-observer variation if one interviewer changed the style of interviewing during the course of the day, perhaps beginning the day interrogating in a leisurely manner and becoming more hurried as the crowds gathered and the day wore on. Observer error may be minimized by careful design and testing of questionnaires (Ch. 6).

The problem of observer variation is well known to the staff of laboratories doing routine medical biochemistry, and elaborate methods have been devised to recognize and correct it so that a laboratory produces standardized results throughout the year. In epidemiological work observer variation can be minimized by careful preliminary training of the survey personnel in the use of the particular technique or questionnaire. Throughout the course of the survey the work must be supervised to ensure that the procedures do not vary from the initial standard. The identity of the observer is an essential part of each recording so that, after completion of the survey, any differences in results obtained by different observers, or by one observer at different times, may be quantified.

Testing the technique

An attribute of an accurate measurement is that it is *repeatable,* i.e. it remains the same when repeatedly elicited. Measurement of a person's height using a satisfactory technique should give a reasonably constant figure irrespective of who does the measurement.

However, many biological phenomena do not remain constant and a single measurement of blood pressure may not be repeatable because the pressure changes from moment to moment. A measurement is not repeatable for one of three reasons: the measuring instrument is intrinsically inaccurate, the phenomenon measured changes, or there is observer variation or error.

When testing a technique an assessment must be made of these three sources of non-repeatability. The method by which this is done depends upon the particular technique but there are certain simple generalizations which apply to all techniques. The limits of accuracy of a measuring instrument and the extent to which any one shows consistent differences from others is determined by comparison of measurements made with different instruments. Assessment of non-repeatability due to variation in the phenomenon being measured must depend upon repeated measurements in the same subject, e.g. haematocrit measurements on samples of blood taken at hourly intervals. Tests of within-observer variation require repeated measurements of the same phenomenon by one observer, e.g. replicate measurements of arm circumference.

Within-observer variation may often be minimized by recording the mean of several replicate measurements rather than using a single measurement. However, between-observer variation is liable to give rise to systematic differences between the observations of different observers and cannot be minimized by an observer repeating the measurements. For example, one observer may consistently record diastolic blood pressure at a higher level than another because he records the level at which the sounds become muffled whereas his colleague records the level at which they disappear. Their results cannot be combined, and will not become more comparable if each makes replicate measurements. Tests of between-observer variation depend upon measurement of the same phenomenon by different observers, for example the weight of an infant being recorded by one observer and then by another.

Sometimes the problems of between-observer variation can be reduced by moving observers from one place to another. In a comparison of the incidence of measles in different villages, recording in each village should optimally be done by more than one observer; each observer should work in more than one village.

The results of repeatability tests of observations on attributes, such as clinical symptoms and signs, are first set out in a table, as illustrated by Table 2.5.

The overall level of agreement could be expressed by $(a + d)$ as

Table 2.5   Results of a repeatability test

| | | Observer 1 | |
		Positive	Negative
Observer 2	Positive	a	b
	Negative	c	d

a proportion of the total. However, this expression, like predictive values, varies according to the actual frequency of the attribute in the group being studied. Repeatability defined as $a/(a + b + c)$ is largely independent of disease frequency. It represents the number of positives agreed by both observers as a proportion of all positives recorded by either observer. An alternative expression $(a + c)/(a + b)$ represents the bias between one observer (or test) and the other.

Repeatability tests on variables such as blood pressure may be summarized by the standard deviation of replicate measures. The standard deviation is a measure of the scatter of observations around their mean, or average, and is described in Chapter 8. For both attributes and variables separate calculations are made for within- and between-observer variation.

The problem of repeatability of measurements in epidemiology always merits careful thought before a survey is begun. It requires reference to publications which describe the techniques and their sources of error. If a new technique is used experimentation is necessary to estimate repeatability and a statistician's assistance is required.

COUNTING DISEASES

In epidemiology various terms are used to describe the frequency with which diseases occur. The purpose of these terms is to allow comparison of disease frequencies in different populations.

The simplest method of expressing disease frequency is a statement of the *number of cases* seen. Thus the WHO recorded 894 cases of AIDS in Brazil during 1986. This defines the burden which AIDS imposed on the health services in Brazil. But comparisons made between the occurrence of the disease in Brazil and in other countries are not very informative unless the size of the population of Brazil in 1986 is also recorded. Therefore statements of disease frequency are usually accompanied by a statement of the number of people in the *related population*. In this way disease frequency is expressed in terms of various rates. The concept of a related population is an important one. Populations may be defined by their location, e.g. the population of Brazil, or may be defined in other terms, e.g. schoolchildren or pregnant women (Ch. 3)

A *rate* may be defined as the number of persons with a disease (or state or event related to a disease) per unit of population per unit of time. To calculate a rate one requires not only the number of people (x) with the disease but also the number (y) who do not have it. The rate is expressed as a ratio of x to ($x + y$). Rates therefore have a numerator (x) and a denominator ($x + y$).

Rates may express *morbidity*, which is the frequency of illness, or *mortality*, the frequency of death. The rates in common use are as follows.

Incidence rates

Incidence may be defined as the frequency of occurrence of some event related to disease, such as onset of symptoms, related to the size of the population and a specified time.

Examples of incidence rates are:

1. The incidence of pulmonary tuberculosis in Tanzania during 1985, as recorded by the WHO, was 4 per 10 000 population. In this example the 'event related to the disease' is its diagnosis.

2. In Vura County, Uganda, between 1956 and 1978, the incidence of hospital admission for schistosomiasis was 7.6 per 10 000 population per year. This incidence rate is derived from the number of events, i.e. admissions for schistosomiasis, and not the number of persons. A person will contribute to more than one event if he or she is admitted with schistosomiasis more than once during the year. In this usage the incidence rate may be referred to as an *admission rate*. Similarly, observation of the number of streptococcal throat infections occurring in a school during a period of time will give an incidence rate which is derived from the number of events, not persons, and may be termed an *attack rate*.

3. The incidence of reported deaths from infective and parasitic diseases in Sri Lanka in 1983 was 48 per 100 000 population. In this example the 'event related to the disease' is death, and this rate is therefore a *death rate*.

Incidence rates are the usual method whereby disease frequency in different populations is compared. Before making such comparisons the rates are usually standardized, to allow for the differing age/sex structure of populations. *Standardization* is described in Chapter 8. Unstandardized rates are referred to as *crude* rates. (It may be noted that the meaning of the word 'standardized' in this context is the same as in the context of standardized procedures for making observations discussed earlier in this chapter. Observations or rates are standardized so that they may be compared with other observations or rates.)

Prevalence rates

By general usage prevalence rates have come to be synonymous with what were otherwise called *point prevalence rates*. They define the proportion of people affected by a disease at one particular time. Thus the prevalence of trachoma recorded during a survey in Iraq in 1975 was 15%. The prevalence rate of a disease is compounded of the incidence rate and the average duration before it is terminated either by recovery or death. During an epidemic cholera may have a very high monthly incidence, but since the course of the disease is usually swift, the prevalence of cases on any one day will be considerably less than this monthly incidence. On the other hand for a chronic disease such as trachoma the annual incidence is much below the prevalence. Where incidence and prevalence are reasonably constant, prevalence can be estimated by the expression:

$$\text{Prevalence} = \text{incidence} \times \text{average duration}$$

Prevalence rates will be altered if people with a disease selectively immigrate into or emigrate from a population. Among schoolchildren, for example, any serious disorder is likely to lead to the withdrawal of a child from school, and consequently the prevalences of diseases are less than those which are predicted from the incidences and durations.

Prevalence rates are administratively useful; but comparison of prevalence rates in different populations is difficult. However, it is frequently easier to measure prevalence rather than incidence since the former can be obtained in a single study (a cross-sectional study), completed within a few weeks, whereas the latter requires accurate ascertainment of the disease over a period of months or years (a longitudinal study). In aetiological studies the incidence is generally more useful than the prevalence, since one is able to use variations in incidence, during different seasons of the year for example, to pinpoint causative influences which operate at the inception of the disease.

Birth and death rates

The *crude birth rate* is usually calculated by relating total live births in a year to the total population. The *crude death rate* is usually calculated by relating total deaths in a year to the total population.

Table 2.6   Annual birth and death rates per 1000 population in selected countries in 1988

Country	Birth rate	Death rate
West Germany	10	11
France	14	10
Japan	11	6
Mauritius	19	7
Pakistan	43	15
Zaire	45	15
Libya	39	8
Kenya	54	13

Table 2.6 shows some striking contrasts in birth and death rates among the countries of the world. Subtraction of the crude death rate from the crude birth rate gives the current annual *growth rate* of a population (exclusive of migration). Growth rates are customarily expressed as percentages and in Table 2.6 they vary from −0.1% in West Germany to +4.1% in Kenya. Growth rates above 3.5% will, if sustained, double the size of a population in less than 20 years.

In many developing countries declining death rates have led to a large difference between birth and death rates, and the resulting high growth rates give so-called 'population explosions'. In Mauritius a malaria control programme began in 1945. By 1962 the death rate had fallen from 27.1 per 1000 to 9.3, but the birth rate had remained at a high level, 38.5. The population of the islands had increased alarmingly, by 50%, and in 1964 it was necessary for the government to implement a major family planning programme. Since then, while the population has continued to increase, the rate of increase has sharply declined.

Analysis of age-specific death rates in most developing countries shows that the highest rates are among young children. For this reason the *life expectancy* at birth, a statistic derived from current age/sex-specific death rates in a population, may be short. The life expectancy at birth in Sierra Leone is quoted as being 35 years. Other examples of life expectancy are shown in Figure 8.10.

Special mortality rates

There are a number of special mortality rates in general use. They are derived from the basic formula for calculation of incidence rates, i.e. number of deaths per unit of population per unit of time.

Included among special mortality rates are the following:

1. The *case fatality rate* is the proportion of persons who die from a disease within a specified time among all those who contract the disease.

During an epidemic of whooping cough in Gulf Province, Papua New Guinea, in 1978 there were 122 patients admitted to hospital of whom 32 died — a case fatality rate of 22%. (This epidemic occurred despite 80% of children being fully immunized: subsequent inquiry revealed that poor refrigeration had reduced the efficacy of the vaccine.)

2. The *infant mortality rate* is the number of infants (children under 1 year old) who died during a year, related to the number of livebirths during the same year. This expression infant deaths/livebirths is multiplied by 1000 so that the infant mortality rate is recorded as the number of infant deaths per 1000 livebirths.

Recently recorded infant mortality rates range from 5.4 per 1000 in Iceland to 175 per 1000 in Mali.

3. The *neonatal mortality rate* is similar to the infant mortality rate: it is the number of children dying in the neonatal period (up to 28 days after birth) during 1 year per 1000 livebirths occurring in the same year.

In many developing countries accurate records of neonatal deaths are difficult to obtain. The 1987 WHO Statistics Annual (one of the series of statistical reports published annually since 1973) records a wide range of neonatal death rates: 17.3 per 1000 in Sri Lanka, 16.9 in Uruguay, 10.1 in Chile. These may be compared with rates of 7.6 per 1000 in the USA and 4.4 in Denmark.

4. The *post-neonatal mortality rates* is the number of children dying in the post-neonatal period (from 4 weeks to 1 year after birth) during 1 year per 1000 livebirths occurring in the same year.

Similarly to neonatal deaths, reliable data are often difficult to obtain. In 1985 the WHO reported rates of 37.3 per 1000 in livebirths in Guatemala to below 5 per 1000 in almost all European countries.

5. The *stillbirth rate* is the number of stillbirths (deaths after the 28th week of pregnancy) occurring during 1 year in every 1000 *total births* (livebirths plus stillbirths). In 1984 the stillbirth rate in Den-

mark was 4.1 per 1000. Stillbirth rates are seldom recorded in developing countries but in 1982 the rate was 10.2 in Malaysia.

6. The *perinatal mortality rate* is the number of stillbirths plus the number of deaths in the first 7 days after birth per year per 1000 total births. It is known that a proportion of deaths which occur within a few days after birth are incorrectly registered as stillbirths, thereby inflating the stillbirth rate and lowering the neonatal mortality rate. The perinatal mortality rate, being a combination of late fetal and early neonatal deaths, is not influenced by this error. Furthermore the two types of death have certain common causes, for example toxaemia and birth trauma.

Because of the difficulties of obtaining accurate data, especially in relation to stillbirths, many countries have no record of prevailing perinatal mortality rates. Those recorded by the WHO in the 1987 Statistics Annual include rates of 19.1 per 1000 in Sri Lanka and 8.4 in the UK.

7. *The maternal mortality rate* is the number of maternal deaths ascribed to puerperal causes per 1000 total births. When stillbirths are not recorded the denominator consists of livebirths only. The 1988 World Health Statistics Annual estimates maternal mortality in Africa to be 640 per 100 000 livebirths whilst it is only 10 per 100 000 in western Europe.

Special rates

Usually rates are calculated by expressing the numbers of cases (the numerator) as a fraction of either the total related population or that section of the population which is *at risk* of the disease (the denominator). Gonorrhoea incidence rates are expressed in relation to the population aged 15 years or more because the disease is unusual in children.

When it is necessary to take account of variations in the intensity or duration of exposure within a population, a denominator may be used other than the related population. When calculating the frequency of industrial disorders the number of person-years worked in the industry gives an incidence rate that reflects the risk of an industrial hazard more precisely than one based on the total number of employed persons. Similarly, in international comparisons of road traffic accidents the numbers of accidents per 1000 vehicles, or per million vehicle miles driven, is a more useful denominator than the total population, of whom many will not use vehicles.

Comparison of rates

When disease frequency in different populations is compared it is essential to ensure that the rates used are comparable. The incidence of tuberculosis in one country cannot be directly compared with the prevalence in another.

3. Populations and samples

POPULATIONS

Throughout this book it is emphasized that a basic requirement in the design of any epidemiological study is a clear definition of its purpose. Consideration of this purpose will usually suggest an approximate definition of the population to be studied, in terms of location and restriction to a particular age-group, sex or occupation. If the purpose of a study is to determine the nutritional status of children in Haiti, then the population must comprise children in Haiti. But this approximate definition will need to be modified, for example by specification of the age limits of children and a decision as to whether to include or exclude recent immigrants.

Use of the word *population* in epidemiology does not correspond with its demographic meaning of an entire group of people living within certain geographical boundaries. A population for an epidemiological study may comprise groups of people defined in many different ways, for example gold mine workers in Africa, children vaccinated against hepatitis B, or pilgrims travelling to Mecca.

It is usually unnecessary as well as impracticable to make observations on an entire population, such as all children in Haiti, since observations made on a properly selected *sample* of appropriate size will enable generalizations to be made about the population. Generalizing from observations made on the nutritional status of a sample of children in Haiti to the nutritional status of all Haitian children is a formalized procedure, in so far as the errors which this may engender can to some extent be specified in advance. However, observations on a study population, such as Haiti, may be used to generalize about nutritional problems in a wider area such as the Caribbean as a whole. Although this may be a reasonable use of the data it is an informal procedure liable to unknown errors, since it is not known to what extent the study population of Haiti is typical of the larger population — that of the Caribbean — to which it belongs.

The problems encountered in defining populations differ for descriptive and analytic studies.

Descriptive studies

In descriptive studies it is usual to define a *study population* and then make observations on a sample taken from it. Study populations are commonly defined by geographical location, age and sex, with additional specification of attributes and variables such as occupation and ethnic group.

Geographical location

In field surveys it is often convenient to use a population defined by an administrative boundary, e.g. a district or a province. This may simplify the problems of enlisting the help of local officials and obtaining the co-operation of the people on whom the investigation will be carried out. In addition data on population size and age/sex structure, derived from official censuses, are usually published according to administrative population groupings. However administrative boundaries do not necessarily define homogeneous groups of people. Since it is often preferable that a single descriptive study does not cover a number of distinct groups of people, with widely differing ways of life or origins, it may be necessary to restrict the study to a particular ethnic group, and thus obtain greater genetic or cultural homogeneity. Alternatively a population may be defined in relation to a prominent geographical feature, such as a river or mountain, which imposes a certain uniformity of behaviour upon the peoples who live near to it.

If cases of a disease are being ascertained through their attendance at a clinic, rather than by field surveys in the community, it will be necessary to define the population according to the so-called *catchment area* of the clinic. For administrative purposes a dispensary, health centre or hospital is usually considered to serve a population within a defined geographical area. But these catchment areas may only accord in a general way with the actual usage of medical facilities by local people.

Catchment areas are profoundly modified by the demography of the area and by the *accessibility* of the clinic or hospital. Accessibility has three aspects — physical, economic and social. It is discussed in more detail in Chapter 11.

Ascertainment of a particular disease within a catchment area may be incomplete either because some patients seek treatment elsewhere, in which case records at neighbouring clinics will reveal this, or more usually because some patients do not seek treatment at all. In the latter case this incomplete ascertainment may be evident from low rates of incidence and prevalence recorded in the area in comparison with rates recorded in other surveys. Discussions with the local people, especially those in one or two of the more remote parts of an area, may quickly reveal whether serious under-ascertainment is occurring.

Where it is impossible to relate cases of a disease to a population, perhaps because the cases were ascertained through a hospital with an indefinable catchment area, *proportional morbidity rates* may be used. These rates have been widely used in cancer epidemiology where the number of cases of one form of cancer is expressed as a proportion of the number of cases of all forms of cancer among patients attending the same hospital during the same period. Clearly this method of expressing disease frequency is liable to errors, for the frequency of one form of cancer may appear to rise or fall solely because of changes in the frequency of other forms of cancer. However, proportional morbidity rates are a convenient method for the initial identification of geographical differences. In one government hospital in East Africa it was noted that 58% of strangulated inguinal hernias were direct compared with 3% in hospitals in the UK. This observation led to the discovery of a remarkably high prevalence of direct inguinal hernias among the population of the area.

Age and sex

The age and sex structure of the study population may be determined by the disease being studied. A survey of carcinoma of the penis, for example, will necessarily be confined to adult males. However, an investigator is often unaware of the age and sex distribution of a disease and must include all age and sex groups in the study population. Sometimes one may choose to limit a study to certain of the age and sex groups affected by a disease. A nutrition survey may be limited to children under 3 years old because nutritional deficiencies are often an especially important health problem in this group.

Occupation

A particular occupational group may be selected for study because of their unusual exposure to a disease, for example fishermen and schistosomiasis. But an occupational group may also be convenient for a study because employees are listed and can easily be organized to attend for interview and examination. In India studies on railway employees have provided interesting data on the distribution of a range of diseases including ischaemic heart disease, peptic ulcer and varicose veins. Medical officers with responsibilities for plantations, factories, refugee settlements and other organizations have exceptional opportunities for epidemiological surveys. However, it is necessary to be cautious when generalizing from observations on an occupational group to the whole population in an area, for occupational groups are usually unrepresentative of all persons in similar age/sex groups. Schoolchildren are convenient and accessible study populations, but many of the poorer children may not attend school and when children at school become ill they tend to discontinue attendance. A study population of schoolchildren is therefore unlikely to be representative of the total population of children, and is not suitable for certain types of study, for example prevalence surveys of heart disease.

Analytic studies

Case-control studies

Whereas in descriptive studies it is usual to define a study population and then make observations on a sample from it, in case-control studies observations may be made on a group of patients, the *study group*, who are not selected by formal sampling of a defined larger group. For instance, a study on patients with deildrin poisoning may include every patient with this diagnosis admitted to one hospital during a certain period of time. However, in such circumstances there is a notional population comprising all patients with the disorder in the particular region or country; although the investigator does not use formal sampling techniques to select the group of patients in the study he is still under an obligation to ascertain the extent to which the group is representative of all patients with the disorder. Studies are often carried out on babies born in hospital because they are a more convenient and accessible group than babies born at home. The two groups of babies differ in many respects, for example those born in hospital tend to come

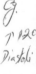

from primiparous mothers and wealthier homes, and at the outset of an investigation it is necessary to determine whether these differences will influence the findings. Generally analytic studies are not carried out on groups of patients who are atypical of all patients with the disorder, unless there is a special indication to do this. An analytic study of viral hepatitis would not be confined to patients who died from the disorder, unless the purpose of the study was to identify the determinants of death in those with the disorder itself. For common diseases such as schistosomiasis formal sampling techniques may be used to select a representative group of cases from among all those known to have the disease.

The choice of cases will require a predetermined definition of what constitutes a case. From clinical practice one gains the impression that a case of disease is clearly defined. Generally there is little problem in deciding whether a patient has or has not got diseases such as diabetes or hypertension, but this is because blood sugar or blood pressure levels need to be greatly raised before sufficient symptoms develop to take a patient to hospital. Figure 3.1 shows the distribution of blood pressure in a population of middle-aged men. The curve is continuous and has only one peak. 'Normotension' merges imperceptibly with 'hypertension', and any definition of an upper level of normal is clearly arbitrary. To a greater or lesser extent almost all diseases are similar to hypertension in having a continuum of severity. Infectious diseases have subclinical as well as clinical forms. Malignant diseases have premalignant forms. The decision as to what is a case must therefore be to some extent arbitary, and it is necessary to use definitions

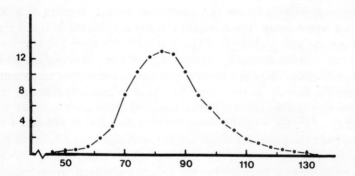

Fig. 3.1 Distribution of diastolic blood pressure in a population of middle-aged men.

which can be precisely described and if possible quantified. Only in this way can the results of one survey be compared with another.

In selecting a study group of cases it is necessary to decide whether to include only newly diagnosed cases or all cases. A disadvantage of using patients with long-standing disease is that their memory of exposure to a suspected determinant before the onset of illness may be inaccurate.

Cohort studies

The principles of a cohort study are described in Chapter 1. In its simplest form its purpose is to compare two groups of individuals, or cohorts, and show whether or not there are more cases of the disease among the cohort exposed to the suspected determinant than among the cohort who are not exposed. In order to establish whether there is an association between forceps delivery and the subsequent development of childhood epilepsy two cohorts are necessary: (1) a study cohort of children born by forceps delivery and (2) a control cohort of children born by uncomplicated deliveries. These two groups of children are followed up for a number of years and cases of epilepsy in either group are recorded. If forceps delivery is associated with the development of epilepsy more cases will occur in group (1) than in group (2). The two most important characteristics of a study cohort are that it should include individuals exposed to the determinant being investigated, and that it should comprise a group of people who can be followed up for the period of time between exposure to the determinant and development of the disorder. It is important that the follow-up of a cohort should be complete or very nearly so. If more than a small proportion of persons in the cohort cannot be traced the observations will be *biased*, or prejudiced, since those untraced are unlikely to be representative of all those in the initial cohort.

According to the kind of determinant being studied there may or may not be a range of choice of cohorts exposed to it. An investigation into the relationship between gold mining and silicosis requires a cohort of people working in gold mines. But an investigation into the association of smoking and lung cancer offers a much wider range of possible cohorts.

The problems associated with making repeated observations on a cohort vary with the length of time over which the investigation extends. In an investigation of bacterial food poisoning the interval of time between ingestion of the infected food and development of gastroenteritis is only a few hours or days, but an investigation into the relationship between hepatitis B infection and the subsequent development of hepatocellular carcinoma must extend over many years. For such prolonged studies it is essential to select a cohort that is (1) stable (not liable to substantial migrations), and will therefore be available for observation over the required period, (2) co-operative and likely to remain so throughout the study and (3) easily accessible to the investigator so that the expense and labour of the study are minimized. Occupational groups, such as members of the armed forces, have obvious advantages for cohort studies. In one investigation a cohort of tsetse control workers provided an ideal cohort for a 3-year study of the relationship between contact with swamps and the development of mycobacterial skin ulcers.

Although a cohort may require observation over a number of years it is not always necessary for the investigator to make these observations prospectively. In a *prospective* cohort study the investigator observes the occurrence of the disease at the time when the cases appear. On the other hand in a *retrospective* cohort study the investigator records the occurrence of the disease a long while after the event. The 3-year survey of mycobacterial skin ulcers already referred to was accompanied by a retrospective survey for 1969 which was carried out in 1970. The camps in which each tsetse control worker had lived during 1969 were recorded in the administrative records; those who developed mycobacterial skin ulcers had been treated at either one of two hospitals, where records were available. It was therefore possible to map those camps where skin ulcers occurred and relate them to the swamps, and in effect, by using accumulated records of both patients and the population, observations on the cohort during 1 year were carried out by the investigator during 2 or 3 days. This retrospective method of doing cohort studies is swift and convenient, but depends upon the availability of complete records. Since the recorded data may not include all that is required retrospective studies may be inaccurate.

SAMPLES

In most surveys it is neither feasible nor necessary to make observations on the entire population being studied, and observations are usually restricted to a sample of individuals. Sampling must be carried out in such a way that it is possible to generalize from the sample to the study population. A number of techniques which achieve this have been devised. Only the simpler techniques will be considered here, but these, used with care, will meet the requirements of many types of study. When more complex sampling methods are needed it may be advisable to enlist the help of a statistician.

Sample size

Observations are made on a sample with the purpose of generalizing from them to the entire study population. The precision with which one can generalize from a sample is related to the size of the sample. Consider a population of 100 000 people among whom the prevalence rate of hookworm infestation is 40%. If a sample of 100 people was selected and examined it is unlikely that the hookworm infestation rate would be exactly 40%. Whatever procedure was used to select the 100 individuals in the sample the operation of chance factors makes it unlikely that the sample would be completely representative of the study population.

Anyone who has gone to a market to buy a sack of grain is familiar with the fundamentals of sampling. The buyer knows that if he examines a handful of grain from the sack it will not be exactly representative of all the grain in the sack. But unless he is unlucky in the particular handful he takes, or unless the seller has deliberately put all the bad grain at the bottom of the sack, he knows that examination of a handful will give a reasonable estimate of the quality of the sackful. Furthermore the more handfuls he examines the more exact will become his estimate of the quality.

An estimate of the hookworm infestation rate in the population derived from observations on a sample will be imprecise. But, providing the technique of sampling is unbiased, the larger the sample the more precise the sample estimate will become. A sample of 1000 people will give a more precise estimate of the hookworm rate than a sample of 100. The final choice of sample size in an investigation is determined by balancing the increased precision given by examining a larger sample against the extra cost and time this will require.

The degree of precision with which measurements in samples of a given size estimate values in the study population may be calculated from simple statistical formulae. The formulae used differ according to whether the observations made are binary — in which only the presence or absence of a characteristic is recorded e.g. the presence or absence of hookworm ova, or quantitative — in which measurements are made on a scale e.g. the haemoglobin concentration in g/100 ml. (The distinction between binary and quantitative data is considered further in Chapter 8.)

Binary data

Observations on the presence or absence of symptoms, signs or other attributes in a sample may be used to estimate disease rates in the study population. The precision of a sample estimate of rates may be specified by the *sampling error*. Suppose that a hookworm infestation rate of 40% is observed in a sample of 100. The formula for calculation of the sampling error of a percentage is $\sqrt{(pq/n)}$ where p = percentage of persons affected, q = percentage of persons not affected, and n = number in sample. The sampling error in the example is therefore $\sqrt{(40 \times 60/100)} \stackrel{\scriptstyle\frown}{=} 5$. According to statistical theory *confidence limits* (for a 95% probability level) are derived by multiplying the sampling error by a factor of approximately 2. The result in this example is 10, which denotes that in 95% of samples of 100 individuals in which a rate of 40% is observed the true rate in the parent population will lie between (40 −10) = 30% and (40 + 10) = 50%. Thus the confidence limits of 30 to 50 define the range of values within which the true population rate will lie for 95% of samples of similar size in which a similar rate is observed. In statistical terms the probability is 95% that the estimate obtained from the sample will not differ from the true rate by more than the range defined by the confidence limits. With increase in sample size the sampling error becomes smaller so that, for example, a hookworm rate of 40% observed in a sample 400 will have confidence limits of only 35 to 45.

It will be noted that the sampling error depends on the prevalence of the condition, so that to obtain a given precision it is necessary to study larger samples for uncommon conditions than for common ones. It can also be seen that sampling error is proportional to the square root of sample size, so that doubling the sample size would only increase precision by a factor of 1.4.

Quantitative data

The values of measurements such as haemoglobin levels or blood pressure will show *variation* among members of a population. This variation has two components: differences in values between one individual and another, and differences in values in one individual at different times. Both of these differences may be distorted — either exaggerated or diminished — by errors in the measurement technique.

For quantitative data the precision of sample estimates may be expressed by the *standard error of the mean* and depends upon the extent of the variation in the measurements made. To obtain a given degree of precision a larger sample is required for variables showing a wide range of values than for those with a lesser range. The standard error (s.e.) is calculated from the expression s.d./ $\sqrt{n}$ where s.d. is the 'standard deviation' of values in the sample and n is the number of individuals in the sample. The standard deviation is a measure of the scatter of observations around their mean, or average, and is described in Chapter 8.

If an investigator is able to make an approximate prediction of the standard deviation of the variable being measured, and can specify the standard error acceptable to him, the expression $n = (s.d./s.e.)^2$ may be used to calculate the required sample size before an investigation is begun. For example, using published data on blood pressure it may be calculated that 95% of samples of 50 subjects will have a mean that is within about 5 mm of the true population mean.

Choice of sample size

By specifying in advance the sampling error (binary data) or standard error (quantitative data) which is acceptable to him an investigator can calculate the size of sample which will give the degree of precision required. However, the dominant considerations in the choice of sample size must often be practical ones such as the availability of time, staff and money. If the investigator's decision about sample size is made solely by reference to practical considerations he will examine as large a sample as is feasible, and must accept whatever error is associated with the resulting sample estimates. In simple descriptive studies this procedure may be satisfactory, although the usefulness of sample estimates associated with large errors may be limited. But in preventive trials (Ch. 10) an investigator who does not consider sampling errors when designing the trial may find at the end that his sample size was too small to reveal effects of the preventive measure which are of public health importance.

Two WHO publications, listed in Suggested Further Reading (p. 169) have tables giving both the size of sample required to achieve a given degree of precision and the precision of estimates derived from a given sample size.

It must be borne in mind that there are many sources of error other than sampling, such as mistakes of measurement, laboratory technique, and non-response of individuals selected for inclusion in a sample. There is little purpose in stipulating a small sampling error if errors from these other sources are likely to be considerable.

Sampling methods

A sample must be selected in such a way that it is possible to generalize from observations made on the sample to the characteristics of the study population. The following methods of sampling are in general use.

Simple random sampling

A sample may be defined as random if every individual in the population being sampled has an equal likelihood of being included. Random selection is the basis of all good sampling techniques, and precludes any method of selection based on volunteering or the choice of groups of people known to be co-operative.

In order to select a *simple random sample* from a population it is first necessary to identify all individuals from whom the selection will be made. In developing countries listings of all persons living in an area are not usually available. If official lists are available, such as taxpayers or census lists, they are likely to be an incomplete representation of the population. People may try to avoid being listed as taxpayers, and when a census is carried out it may be difficult to identify all members of nomadic communities or groups of individuals such as fishermen whose occupation takes them away from home. Whether or not defects in official lists make them invalid for epidemiological purposes depends upon the particular investigation being carried out. To make a complete listing of a study population for the purposes of a single survey is usually too laborious and time-consuming. Two-stage sampling (see p. 39) will greatly reduce this task and make it feasible.

The usual method of selecting a simple random sample from a listing of individuals is to assign a number to each individual and then select certain numbers by reference to random number tables, which are published in books of statistical tables such as that of Lindley & Scott (see Suggested Further Reading, p. 170).

Systematic sampling

An alternative method of sampling is to take a *systematic sample*, in which every *nth* person is selected from a list or from some other ordering. A systematic sample can be drawn from a queue of people, or from patients ordered according to the time of their attendance at a clinic. Thus a sample can be drawn without an initial listing of all persons among whom the selection will be made. In this a systematic sample has a major practical advantage over a simple random sample.

In order to fulfil the statistical requirements for a random sample a systematic sample should be drawn from patients who are randomly ordered. The starting point for selection should be randomly chosen. If every third person on a register is being selected then a random procedure must be used to determine whether the first, second or third person on the register is chosen as the first member of the sample. Clearly there are three possible samples: (1) patients 1, 4, 7 . . . (2) patients 2, 5, 8 . . . (3) patients 3, 6, 9 . . .

In practice the ordering of individuals from whom a systematic sample is selected is not usually random. However, this imperfect randomization may usually be disregarded in surveys but prohibits systematic sampling in trials (Chapter 10).

Multi-stage sampling

In a survey covering a district, province or country an initial sample may be taken from units of the population such as villages. The villages are listed and a random sample of the required number selected. Then a listing of individuals within the chosen villages is made and a sample taken from them. This is two-stage sampling which was used, for example, in the WHO tuberculin surveys in Africa. The same procedure of subdividing the population into progressively smaller units may be extended to three or more stages as required. This method of sampling has the advantage that a listing of persons is only required for the relatively small unit from which the final selection is made. If the initial subdivisions of the population are made on the basis of geographical distribution the resulting sample, for example a number of villages, is a *cluster* sample, so called because the individuals selected are clustered in one place. In field surveys it is obviously convenient to use a sample of people who all live in the same area. When cluster samples are small units of the population, such as villages, clans or families, it may simplify the fieldwork if all individuals in the clusters are included in the study rather than a sample of them. The members of a household often find it difficult to comprehend why the doctor is visiting the home next door but not visiting them.

Cluster sampling of a population is liable to cause errors if the disease, attribute or variable being studied is itself clustered in the population. Cases of onchocerciasis may be clustered around streams suitable for the breeding of *Simulium* flies. In an area away from the streams the villages may contain no cases, whereas in an area close to streams almost every person may be affected. The selection of five villages as cluster samples to show the prevalence of onchocerciasis in a district may give misleading results. By chance the selected villages may be quite unrepresentative of the entire population in the proportion of villages 'exposed' to onchocerciasis and 'not exposed.' One might, by chance, select five villages which are all close to streams, and thereby infer that more than 90% of the district population was affected. Alternatively five villages away from streams could be selected and the inference made that the disease did not occur in the district. To avoid such difficulties it is necessary to carry out an initial survey, and establish the degree of clustering before taking cluster samples.

Stratified sampling

If a disease is unevenly distributed within a population in respect of sex, age, or some other attribute or variable it may be better to choose a stratified sample. To obtain a sample stratified by age, for example, the study population is subdivided into age-groups, such as 0–14 years, 15–49, and 50 and over. A different fraction of each age-group is then selected as the sample, either by simple random sampling or systematic sampling. If a disease declines in frequency with increasing age then in order to include in the sample sufficient numbers of cases among older people one might, for example, select from the study population 1 in 8 of the 0–14 years group, 1 in 6 of the 15–49 years group, and 1 in 4 of the 50 and over group.

Choice of sampling method

The choice of a particular sampling method is largely determined by practical considerations. In fieldwork it is almost impossible to select a sample that is fully random. Every sample is therefore to some extent biased and in order to assess this bias the investigator must have some basic knowledge of the study population. A list of taxpayers may be considered adequate for a survey if comparison of numbers of taxpayers with numbers in an official census shows that only a small percentage of the population is avoiding tax. The effort involved in tracing a few tax dodgers to reduce the bias in a sample survey of tuberculin reaction may be quite unrewarding. On the other hand the prevalence of trachoma could not be determined solely by examination of a sample of people attending a health centre. The bias in such a sample could not be predicted by someone working in the health centre, for either trachoma patients might be more willing to attend the centre than those with no visual defects, or trachoma patients, because of their visual defect, might be prevented from finding their way to the centre.

4. Controls

In analytic studies there are usually two groups of individuals. The *study group* comprises persons either affected by a disease (in case-control studies) or exposed to a suspected determinant (in cohort studies). The *control group* comprises persons either unaffected by the disease (in case-control studies) or not exposed to the determinant (in cohort studies).

The selection of study groups and cohorts is discussed in Chapter 3. Selection of control groups and cohorts is an exacting procedure which requires careful thought. If the controls are inappropriate the results of an investigation are of little value.

There are two general principles which govern the choice of controls. Firstly the control group must resemble the study group in certain specified characteristics. Secondly observations made on the control group must be directly comparable to those made on the study group.

CONTROLS IN CASE-CONTROL STUDIES

Consider a specific problem. An investigation is required to show whether hepatitis B virus carriage is sometimes a determinant of hepatocellular carcinoma. In a case-control study an association between virus carriage and cancer will be demonstrated by observation of a higher frequency of hepatitis B carriage among a group of patients suffering from hepatoma than among a group of people without cancer.

In case-control studies the controls differ from the cases primarily in that they are unaffected by the disease. In a study of hepatoma there should be little difficulty in identifying groups of people without the disorder. However, with a disease such as chronic hepatitis, which can have a high incidence in a population and occurs in subclinical forms where diagnosis is difficult, identification of groups of people without the disorder may require special care.

Apart from problems of case definition, which are discussed on page 34, the choice of controls is a critical exercise because of two characteristics shown by many disease determinants.

1. *Exposure to a determinant does not always result in development of a disease.* If hepatitis B carriage invariably led to hepatoma, the selection of controls would present little difficulty. Whatever group of people without hepatoma was used as a control none would be carriers of the hepatitis B virus compared with x% of hepatoma patients.

2. *The frequency of exposure to a determinant varies among different subgroups of a population.* In Africa the prevalence of hepatitis B carriage is lower in urban populations than in rural ones. Household crowding, exposure to blood-sucking arthropods and traditional scarring practices are all less in urban populations and this may explain the differences in carriage.

Consider a second problem. Suppose a doctor in a clinic becomes aware that he has recently been consulted by a number of men with the same complaint of an irritating papular rash on the limbs and trunk. The doctor has been unable to diagnose the condition but recalls that an unusual number of the patients have been immigrants, and not part of the local population. Using his clinic records he carries out a simple case-control study to confirm this observation. Out of 24 patients he has seen with the skin disease (the study group) 18 (75%) are recorded as being immigrants. Out of 220 men with other diseases attending the clinic during the same period (the control group) 44 (20%) are immigrants. Having demonstrated an association between the disease and immigrants he carries out a second case-control study, also using the clinic records. The purpose of this second study is to determine whether the disease tends to occur in immigrant men because of the types of occupation they undertake, since it is known that the immigrants generally do unskilled labouring jobs which the local people are unwilling to do. Of the 18 immigrant patients with the skin disease (the study group) 16 (90%) are recorded as working in the docks. Of the 44 immigrant men with other diseases (the control group) 9 (20%) work in the docks. The skin disease therefore seems to be associated with working in the docks; one may imagine that subsequent investigation of the working habits of the dockers showed that they frequently handled copra infested with mites which transferred themselves to the workers and caused the rash.

This simplified example shows how two different associations are revealed by the use of two different control groups. Clearly, before the control group is selected the objective of the study must be precisely specified.

This can be illustrated by the design of case-control studies to determine risk factors for cerebral malaria. One can envisage a chain of events in malaria infection:

1. Healthy child
   ↓
2. Asymptomatic parasitaemia
   ↓
3. Symptomatic parasitaemia
   ↓
4. Cerebral malaria

If children suffering from cerebral malaria (4) are the cases, controls might be selected to be 1, 2 or 3. If healthy children (1) were the controls then the study would reflect risks of infection as well as those of severe disease. If parasitaemic, symptom-free children (2) were the controls then the study would determine risks of clinical disease of any severity. Whereas if children with symptoms of malaria (3) were used then the question would be specifically about risks of severe versus mild disease. Ideally one might have three control groups to attempt to answer all these questions.

Now consider again the hypothetical example of a case-control study designed to show whether hepatitis B carriage and hepatoma are associated. Suppose that the carriage rate in a certain rural area is 5% whereas, for reasons already suggested, it is lower in the adjacent urban area, 1%. Suppose also that a control group a group of 100 people is required to match with a group of 100 hepatoma patients. If 75 of the controls come from the urban area and 25 from the rural area their carriage rate will be $(75 \times 1 + 25 \times 5)/100 = 2\%$. If the figures are reversed so that 25 of the controls come from the urban area and 75 from the rural area the carriage rate will be $(25 \times 1 + 75 \times 5)/100 = 4\%$. Thus the carriage rate in the controls is doubled merely by selecting them in a different rural:urban ratio. Consequently the comparison between the carriage rate in the control group and that in the cases will be markedly influenced by the rural:urban ratio of the controls.

In this example area of residence is seen as a variable which influences exposure to the suspected determinant. All such variables must be considered during selection of controls and a decision taken as to whether or not the patients and controls should be *matched* in respect of them, so that their influence is nullified. In making this decision a distinction must be made between variables which are associated with both the suspected determinant and the disease and those which are associated with the suspected determinant only. In order to look at this more closely a third example may be used.

Suppose that an investigator wishes to use the case-control method to discover whether women using oral contraceptives are more liable to HIV infection. He will need to identify a study group of female patients with HIV infection and compare the proportion who take oral contraceptives with the proportion in a control group of women not infected with HIV. There are a number of variables which influence whether or not women use contraceptives. On the one hand there are variables such as age which influence both the use of oral contraceptives and the frequency of HIV infection: these are known as *confounding variables*. On the other hand there are variables such as religious belief which have a profound influence on the acceptability and use of oral contraceptives but are generally unlikely to influence the frequency of HIV infection. The principles of matching, whose detailed exposition is beyond the compass of this book, require that an attempt is made to match the patients and controls in respect of all confounding variables but not in respect of variables which influence the suspected determinant alone. If the effect of confounding variables is not neutralized by matching the results of the study may be impossible to interpret. For example the study might show that a higher proportion of the patients with HIV infection used oral contraceptives than did the controls, but if there was no matching on age this result could arise solely because women not using family planning methods were generally younger than those who were using them, and being younger were less likely to be infected with HIV. However, matching on variables such as religious belief would tend to conceal any association between oral contraceptives and HIV infection. In an extreme case perfect matching on every influence which determines the use of oral contraceptives would result in the frequency of their use in the patient and control groups becoming identical. This is *over-matching*.

A kind of variable which has not yet been considered comprises those associated with the development of the disease but not with exposure to the suspected determinant. Genital ulceration, for example, may increase the frequency of HIV infection but probably does not often influence whether a woman takes oral contraceptives. Matching on such variables is generally ineffective as it is of no consequence to the validity of the case-control comparison.

Matching of cases and controls may be accomplished either by stratification of the controls, or by pairing. Stratification of a source of controls into age-groups, for example, and subsequent selection of different proportions of individuals from each strata can be used to give a control group whose age distribution matches that of the cases. In *pairing* a control is selected to pair with a given patient, being identical to the patient in respect of age and other confounding variables. Whichever method is used some degree of protection against errors in matching is afforded by the use of several controls for each case.

In practice it is inpossible to meet the theoretical requirement of matching on all confounding variables. There is unlikely to be sufficient knowledge at the outset of an investigation to enable such variables to be identified; the numbers of potential controls may be limited so that the constraints of rigorous matching criteria lead to insufficient controls being available. However, the investigator must endeavour to assemble a control group which is matched at least in respect of the dominant known confounding variables. Sometimes if individual matching is restricted to the dominant confounding variables it is possible to allow for other variables by group matching or stratification during the analysis. At other times analysis may reveal confounding variables which can only be matched out by design and execution of a further study.

Sources of controls

In selecting individuals as controls the over-riding requirements are to achieve the necessary similarities between cases and controls, in accordance with the principle already defined, and to ensure that observations on the controls are made under the same conditions as those on the cases.

The possible sources from which controls may be selected for case-control studies include hospital patients, relatives, neighbours and the general population.

Hospital patients

Since many case-control studies depend upon investigation of

groups of patients attending a hospital it is often convenient to select a control group from among other patients in the same hospital.
For instance, the socioeconomic background of a group of patients
with viral hepatitis admitted to a hospital in Ghana was compared
with that of a control group drawn from all patients with diseases
other than hepatitis admitted to the same hospital. Since both cases
and controls were in hospital, interviews with both groups were
held under the same conditions, thereby satisfying the second of
the two requirements defined above.

However, the selective process which results in sick people
reaching hospital may differ for different diseases. In a large general
hospital in a city, admission for measles may tend to be restricted
to the more severe cases occurring in the immediate urban
neighbourhood, since it may be difficult for seriously ill children
living further away to undertake the journey. However, children
being treated for chronic osteomyelitis may come from all parts of
the city and the adjacent rural area. Therefore it would be inappropriate to compare the socioeconomic status of measles and
osteomyelitis patients because they would differ merely because of
the different proportions of cases admitted from urban and rural
areas. This can be partly overcome by matching, or stratifying in
the analysis, on district of residence of the patients.

Usually it is unwise to choose a control group from a group of
patients with one disease. In a study of psychosomatic influences
as determinants of heart disease the control group comprised patients with fractures. The study failed to show an association between psychosomatic influences and heart disease because these
influences proved to be more important in the aetiology of fractures
(presumably because people with certain psychological characteristics are more prone to accidents). It is even possible that this study
could have wrongly shown that psychosomatic influences protect
against heart disease. Difficulties of this kind may be avoided by
selecting controls who have a range of different disorders.

Relatives

The relatives of individuals affected by a disease may form an appropriate and accessible group from which controls may be selected. Relatives have genetic similarity and tend to share a similar
environment (although in discussion of 'relatives' it must be borne
in mind that the word is loosely used in many societies). Consider
a study whose purpose is to show whether kwashiorkor leads to

subsequent intellectual impairment. In principle such a study seeks to show whether, if a particular group of children had not suffered from kwashiorkor, their measured intelligence would have been higher. But the development of intelligence is subject to numerous genetic and environmental influences, and it is critical to select a control group whose level of intelligence reflects that which would be expected of the group of children who suffered from kwashiorkor. The disease tends to occur in poor families where the general level of education and measured intelligence is low. Clearly it would be inappropriate to compare the intelligence of children from these families with that of children from families on a government housing estate. Comparison with a control group drawn from the families of neighbours would also be misleading because, within a community where kwashiorkor occurs, those families who do not suffer from it may have a slightly higher level of education and intelligence than those in which it occurs. Resolution of this difficulty lies in the use of a control group comprising the brothers and sisters of the patients, since their exposure to the influences determining intelligence will have been more similar to that of the patients than will that of any other group.

The use of relatives as controls has the practical advantages that relatives are usually easily located from information given by the patients, and they are usually willing to co-operate since a member of their family has received medical care. However, in an inquiry into peoples' activities or attitudes, it may be difficult to obtain information from relatives which is comparable to that obtained from the patients if the latter are interviewed while they are in hospital. Patients in hospital who are unwell, removed from their families, and perhaps frightened, may give answers to questions about their activities and attitudes which are different from those they would give were they at home. It is preferable to interview patients at home after their discharge from hospital, so that interviews with patients and controls are conducted under comparable conditions.

There are circumstances when the use of relatives as controls is inappropriate. In an analysis of the influences which determine exposure to *Schistosoma mansoni* infestation, comparison of the activities of patients with the disease and those of relatives without it may be uninformative. In an area where the disease occurs it is likely that all persons are exposed to the parasite and that the occurrence of the disease depends on influences such as the degree of exposure and immunity. Comparison of patients' activities with those of relatives may therefore be relevant to the question 'Among those exposed to the parasite, what determines whether one individual develops the disease while another does not?' but is less relevant to the question 'What determines whether an individual is exposed to the parasite?' Epidemiology is often more successful in answering the second question than the first.

Neighbours

People living in households near to that of a patient offer a control group who share a similar environment but do not have the genetic resemblance of close relatives. In studies of inherited disorders, such as sickle cell disease, this lack of genetic resemblance may be pertinent to their selection as controls.

The use of neighbours as controls tends to require much fieldwork in locating the appropriate persons and sometimes waiting hours for them to return from a market or some other domestic duty. It is important to remember that in selection of controls from neighbours, or any other source, a given individual cannot be discarded in favour of another because he or she is temporarily unavailable. Such a procedure would bias selection towards those neighbours who remain at home throughout the day, perhaps because they are old, infirm, or rich. This is less of a problem with young children, who normally spend all day at home.

The general population

When the required information is recorded for all individuals then the total population may be used as a control group. For example, extensive studies of congenital malformations have been carried out using obstetric data recorded for all 200 000 births occurring in the city of Birmingham, UK, during a 10-year period. This kind of population data is generally unavailable in developing countries. The value of total population data in case-control studies is not that it enables comparison of, for example, the obstetric histories of patients with congenital dislocation of the hip and those of the whole population, but rather that during analysis a comparison may be made between the patients and population data standardized for all confounding variables. The process of standardizing population data is equivalent to selecting the appropriate control group from the population; and the possession of total population data effectively permits the selection of an endless series of control groups for whom the required information is immediately available.

If the relevant data are not recorded for the total population they must be obtained from observations on a sample, taking into account the confounding variables for which cases and controls must be matched. Sampling a population and then making the necessary observations is often time-consuming and expensive. A group of controls selected from a population may be unco-operative, since they will have no personal involvement with the patients in the study, either as fellow hospital patients, relatives, or neighbours.

CONTROLS IN COHORT STUDIES

In a cohort study the frequency of disease in the study cohort exposed to the determinant is compared with that among a cohort with no exposure, or perhaps with a lesser degree of exposure.

The dominant requirements in the selection of controls for cohort studies are twofold.

Firstly, the distribution of the controls must be the same as that of the study cohort in respect of any variable or attribute, other than the suspected cause, which influences the frequency of the disease (rather than in respect of any variable or attribute which influences both exposure to the suspected cause and the frequency of the disease, as in case-control studies).

Secondly, observations on the controls must be made under the same conditions as those on the study cohort. If observations are made on two occupational groups, one of which is serving as the control, difficulties may result from the different levels of medical supervision to which different occupational groups are exposed. Employees of large international mining companies may have routine medical checks, such as X-rays. Roadworkers may be without any form of medical care.

The sources of control data in cohort studies are a separate control cohort, or individuals within the study cohort who do not share the same degree of exposure as other members of the cohort, or national statistics.

Control cohort

The sources of control cohorts include those for case-control studies, i.e. hospital patients, relatives, neighbours, and the general population.

On the one hand hospital patients will often have an altered morbidity and mortality because of the illness that took them to hospital. Healthy relatives and neighbours on the other hand should reflect the general disease experience of the community clearly. They must not be exposed to the possible determinant.

Total populations are often used as controls in cohort studies in developing countries. Where the outcome has a high incidence, and there is a short interval between exposure and disease, a study can be rapidly carried out. For example, in a study of the use of bednets in the prevention of malaria whole villages were studied. Children could be categorized as to whether they slept under a bednet or not. In one rainy season the incidence of malaria as determined by weekly temperature, and blood films from those who were pyrexic, showed a lower incidence of malaria in bednet users. The cause and effect of this association are discussed further in Chapter 10.

Individuals with varying degrees of exposure

Not all members of a cohort, such as an occupational group, may be exposed to a particular hazard. In a study of 22 000 Chinese civil servants about 20% were hepatitis B carriers. All civil servants received similar medical care under the Government insurance scheme and so the 80% who were non-carriers acted as controls for the carriers. Comparison within this cohort was early evidence for the relation between hepatitis B and hepatoma.

National statistics

In developing countries national health statistics are usually inadequate for use as control data. When available such statistics enable the disease experience of a cohort, such as the incidence of bladder carcinoma among workers in the chemical industry, to be compared with the incidence among all members of the population. Such a comparison between disease incidence in a cohort and in the population would require preliminary standardization to allow for the differing distribution of age, sex, and other variables and attributes which influence disease frequency. A difficulty in using national statistics as control data for cohorts of workers is that people do not enter employment if they are ill and leave it if they become ill. The overall health of working people is therefore better than that of the general population — although the rates of the particular diseases associated with an occupation will of course be higher.

Some developing countries have national registers of cancer and if exposures are geographically limited, as for example with

Schistoma haematobium in West Africa, then geographical groups can be examined, with suitable standardization, for evidence of the effects of exposure on cancer. Urinary tract cancer might be examined in this way and the subsequent effects of schistosomiasis control examined by registration rates in successive generations.

5. Some important epidemiological variables and attributes

The distribution of a disease is described in terms of the personal characteristics of those affected, for example their sex and occupation, together with the variations in disease occurrence in different places and at different times. This chapter gives an account of the attributes and variables which are basic to epidemiological distributions of a wide range of diseases. It omits others which are applicable to a restricted range of diseases, for example the immunity of individuals to infections, patterns of agriculture, or the occurrence of animal reservoirs of parasitic disease.

Description of the distribution of a disease leads to an attempt to interpret the distribution in relation to known or suspected determinants. It is helpful to consider determinants under three headings

1. *Host* determinants, e.g. age, occupation, habits.
2. *Agent* determinants, e.g. pathogenicity, dosage, infectivity.
3. *Environmental* determinants, e.g. climate, vector ecology, availability of food.

Interpretation of a distribution may be profoundly modified if the disease occurs frequently in a subclinical and often undiagnosed form, as in viral hepatitis.

AGE

Age is one of the most important variables analysed in epidemiological surveys, and yet it is one of the most difficult to obtain with accuracy in developing countries, where there is often no birth registration and where a considerable proportion of the population may be illiterate. Sometimes records of age may be obtained from government census records, health patrol records, tax census forms, maternal and child health records (usually kept only for very young children), and mission baptismal records (often accurate to the day). Sometimes chiefs, priests, schoolteachers or other prominent people are able to verify the accuracy of people's stated ages.

As with other variables, age must be defined. Therefore it is usual to specify whether age is taken as age at last birthday or next birthday, and whether data on age have been obtained from a precise source, such as a birth certificate, or from some other source such as the average of the person's stated age and the observer's estimate of the age.

Children

Age determination presents the greatest difficulty during nutrition work in young children, when accuracy is required to within a few weeks. Sometimes an estimate of children's ages may be obtained by questioning the mothers about the time of birth in relation to agricultural rhythms and rainfall seasons. Birth ranking within the family may be useful. The timing of primary dental eruption seems little influenced by protein–calorie malnutrition of mild or moderate severity; and unless severe protein–calorie malnutrition is widespread in a community the age of children from 6 to 24 months may be determined for epidemiological (but not clinical) purposes by the formula:

$$\text{age (months)} = 6 + \text{number of erupted teeth}$$

Signs of puberty are useful only as approximate indices of age, because there is much variation between individuals within a population and from one population to another.

Adults

For adults it is usually necessary to get only an approximation of age, and this can often be obtained by referring to a calendar of notable events. By asking people whether they were born or reached puberty before or after the coronation of a king, or the death of a public figure, approximate ages can often be deduced. Other notable events include earthquakes, famines, the 1918 influenza epidemic, world wars, local wars, the building of a railway, a coup d'état, or independence from colonial regimes.

In societies where age at marriage is relatively stable an

adult's age can be deduced from the ages of the children and grandchildren.

Age-groups

The inaccuracies of age determination make small age-groupings inappropriate. The WHO has suggested the following classifications of populations by age-groups for different purposes:

1. To categorize the demographic characteristics of a population three broad groups are useful: 0–14 years, infants and children; 15–49 years, young people and adults; 50 and over, the aged.

2. For morbidity recording five groups may be used: less than 1 year; 1–4 years; 5–14 years; 15–49 years; 50 and over.

3. For detailed studies 14 groups may be used: less than 1 year; 1–4; 5–9; 10–14; 15–19; 20–24; 25–29; 30–34; 35–39; 40–44; 45–49; 50–54; 55–59; 60 and over.

Because of the inaccuracy of recorded ages they are usually grouped in decades, when the groups should be 15–24; 25–34; etc. in order to minimize errors which result when inexactly known ages are rounded off to a multiple of 10.

Age distribution of diseases

Changes in disease frequency at different ages may be represented by histograms or frequency polygons (Ch. 8) in which the frequency of the disease is plotted on the vertical axis and age on the horizontal axis.

Clearly the age distribution of a disease will be influenced by the particular stage of the disease at which it is recorded. The age distributions of primary and tertiary syphilis are very different. Age distributions are also influenced by three factors — population structure, levels of ascertainment and diagnostic criteria.

Population structure

When describing the age distribution of a disease it is important to distinguish between disease frequency expressed *as numbers of cases* and disease frequency expressed as *rates*. Figure 5.1 shows the numbers of new cases of primary liver cancer in The Gambia from 1986 to 1988. The greatest number of cases occurred in the age-group 35–44 years with fewer cases at older ages. Figure 5.2 shows

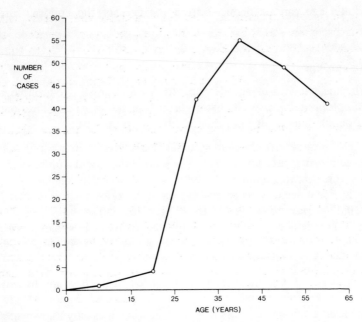

Fig. 5.1 Numbers of new cases of primary liver cancer in The Gambia from 1986 to 1988.

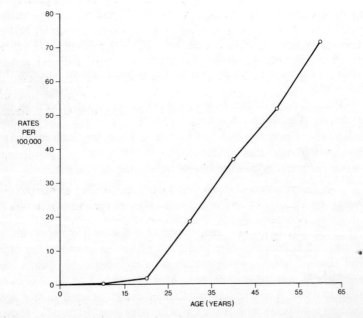

Fig. 5.2 Age-specific incidence rates of primary liver cancer in The Gambia form 1986 to 1988.

the same data expressed as rates. The incidence rises steeply with increasing age and is highest in the oldest age-group. Therefore, as would be expected, the elderly are at greatest risk of death from the disease, but since their numbers in the population are relatively few, they contribute only a small number of deaths to the total. A clinician's experience of the age association of a disease is based on the age distribution of cases. But for investigation of disease determinants it is the incidence curve, reflecting the risk of disease in each age-group, which must be considered.

Levels of ascertainment

The numbers of recorded cases of a disease in each age-group may be influenced by differing use of medical services at different ages. For instance, old people may prefer traditional medicines or may be unable to walk long distances to a clinic; in these circumstances ascertainment of disease among them will be less complete than among younger people.

Diagnostic criteria

Old people are often unwilling to submit themselves to prolonged investigations and their illnesses may be diagnosed less accurately than those of young people. Diagnostic techniques differ for different age-groups. It is, for example, difficult to detect whooping cough or diagnose congenital heart disease in the first year of life. If at certain ages there are differences in diagnostic techniques, or in the individual's willingness to submit to them, or in the doctor's willingness to use them, the recorded age distribution of a disease may be a distortion of the true one.

Interpretation of age distributions

The age distribution of disease incidence may reflect either the differing experiences of different age-cohorts within the population or an association between the disease and changes which occur in individuals as a result of ageing.

Age-cohorts

Within a population people of approximately the same age form an age-cohort, who share a similar environment from birth to death. Consider a population in which a successful yaws eradication programme was carried out in 1940. A prevalence survey carried out in 1980 would show that no person under the age of 40 had the stigmata of yaws, whereas among those over 40 stigmata would be found. This observation is open to the interpretation that yaws does not affect people under 40. But the correct interpretation would clearly lie in the different exposure to yaws of age-cohorts who grew up either before or after the eradication programme.

When studying the age distribution of a disease it is necessary to bear in mind that people in different age-groups differ not only with respect to their current age but also in the environments to which they have been exposed throughout their lives. A disease with a high frequency among young people may be one whose incidence in the population is currently increasing, and a disease with a high frequency among old people may have recently declined in incidence.

Association with ageing

At each age changing biological or behavioural influences alter the patterns of diseases to which people are liable.

Children lack immunity to infection and therefore have a high frequency of diseases such as measles and poliomyelitis. They are liable to kwashiorkor and other nutritional disorders because of the nutritional demands of growth and the hazards imposed by weaning. Their small size makes them more prone to conditions such as dehydration from diarrhoea, or anaemia from hookworm. Their inexperience leads to accidents and trauma. They manifest the results of intrauterine exposure to noxious influences such as the rubella virus or X-rays.

Young adults may be exposed to disease through their occupations. Women are at risk from the large number of disorders associated with reproduction.

Old age brings special stresses from poverty, isolation, malnutrition and bereavement. The cumulative effect of environmental exposures, to alcohol for example, may result in disease. Older people manifest diseases such as tertiary syphilis in which there is a long latent period between exposure and development of signs and symptoms.

SEX

As with age, the sex distribution of a disease may be influenced by the three factors — population structure, levels of ascertainment, and diagnostic criteria.

Population structure

Although the sex ratio at birth is almost equal (103 males : 100 females in Africa), preferential immigration or emigration by one or other sex may lead to considerable imbalance in the total population. In rural eastern Nigeria it has been found that seasonal migration causes cyclic changes in the sex ratio, which rises from 68 males : 100 females in April to 86 : 100 in August. Figure 5.3 shows the age–sex structure of the population of the United Arab Emirates. There is a marked excess of men over women. Almost all of the excess is in the age range 15 to 55 years. It reflects the large numbers of men who have come to work in the United Arab Emirates, leaving their families in their country of origin.

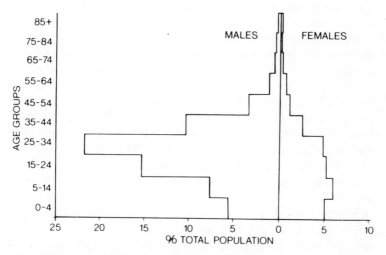

Fig. 5.3 Age–sex structure of the population of United Arab Emirates, 1977 (source: Statistical Agenda, 1978, UAE Ministry of Planning).

Levels of ascertainment

The use made of medical facilities, and consequently the level of ascertainment of disease, may differ for the two sexes. In many communities the women's duties around the house and in the fields make it more difficult for them than for men to spare time to seek medical treatment. Parents may value children of one sex more highly, and be more willing to seek treatment for them.

Diagnostic criteria

Some diseases, such as gonorrhoea, are more difficult to diagnose in one sex than the other. This will influence the recorded incidence in the two sexes.

Interpretation of sex distributions

Variations in disease frequency between the sexes can be due to physiological or other intrinsic differences (as is seen in cancer of the breast), or to behavioural differences. Generally women and girls lead different lives from men: they hoe; they cook; they look after children. They less frequently take part in activities such as hunting and travelling. The extent of role differentiation in the sexes differs between cultures: for instance, in some parts of Africa women go fishing and in other parts they do not. Some differences between the sexes, for example in occupation or exposure to animals, are readily apparent, but differences in such things as food taboos and use of traditional medicines are less obvious.

Kuru, which has been the subject of intensive epidemiological investigation, provides an interesting example of a sex difference in disease frequency. Women were found to be affected more frequently than men, but among children both sexes were affected with equal frequency. The disease has been attributed to a slow virus; it seems likely that the sex pattern of incidence resulted from transmission of the slow virus during the preparation of dead bodies for ritual cannibalistic rites of mourning. These preparations were carried out by women and young children but not by men.

In North America and Europe the overall mortality rates at every age are higher for men than women. By contrast women have higher morbidity rates than men. These sex differences suggest either that women fall ill more commonly than men, but that the diseases which affect them are less often fatal than those which affect men, or that men are less willing to seek medical treatment for minor illnesses. The extent of similar sex differences in mortality and morbidity in developing countries is not known.

ETHNIC GROUP

Ethnic groups have been defined as 'a social group characterised by a distinctive social and cultural tradition, maintained within the group from generation to generation, a common history and origin, and a sense of identification with the group. Members of the group have distinctive features in their way of life, shared experiences, and often a common genetic heritage' (Last J. M., see Suggested Further Reading, p. 169). People in an ethnic group may be similar in diverse ways, for example in birthplace, religion, food habits or enzyme deficiencies. Such characteristics may affect the frequency of disease. Penile cancer, for example, is rare in communities which practise circumcision, and cysticerosis is rare among vegetarians.

The word *tribe* is imprecise, for some tribes are distinguished mainly by their place of residence whereas for others the distinction may be one of language, diet or some other aspect of culture. *Race* is also an imprecise word and carries with it political overtones. Its current usage is certainly not confined to groups of people with a common genetic inheritance and it has no place in scientific writing. *Ethnic group* is more precise and less emotive.

Culture may be defined as an acquired or learned and systematized pattern of behaviour held in common by an organized group of society. Not all aspects of this behaviour pattern apply to every individual. Some elements such as housing, reactions to illness, and language are more or less universal, but there are also specialities, alternatives and individual peculiarities.

The epidemiologist may have to study the *diet* and *food habits* of an ethnic group, perhaps to determine whether the diet is deficient in certain nutrients at certain times of life, or whether there are toxic substances in the food. A rough but easily obtained broad-spectrum view of foods consumed at different ages can be obtained by asking a sample of the population what food was consumed on the previous day. Rates of usage for each food in each age-group can then be established and will indicate which foods are used by all people and which are seldom used. Influences which determine the dietary pattern, such as availability of foods and local customs, may then be discovered by further questioning. It is necessary to bear in mind that variations in diet occur at different times of the year, for instance with religious observances, celebrations, ceremonies or agricultural seasons.

MARITAL STATUS

In developing countries categories such as single, married, widowed, separated are not always precise. The age at marriage may be very young; the degree of cohabitation may vary (for example in parts of New Guinea men live separately from their wives); and 'marriage' may have different meanings depending on religious, social, economic or legal recognition. However, on the whole the married, the single, the widowed and the separated have different ways of life that may be causally related to certain disorders such as venereal disease or nutritional deficiencies. On the other hand the presence of disease may itself determine marital status. People with leprosy and epilepsy tend to remain unmarried or, if they develop the disease while married, they may become divorced or separated. Occupation and socioeconomic status are also related to marital status in societies with high bride prices. Among cattle-keeping peoples who demand many cattle as bride price only the wealthy or those in remunerative employment are able to marry at an early age.

FAMILY STRUCTURE

Leprosy, tuberculosis, trachoma, scabies, tinea and hookworm are among the diseases which may affect many members of a family; family size and the extent of interaction within families has to be considered in the investigation and treatment of many communicable diseases. In countries with extended families the number of individuals living together in a shared habitat, and therefore at risk from communicable diseases, is much greater than in the small nuclear families seen in the cities of industrialized countries. In some developing countries it is not uncommon to find a man and his wives, and his brothers and their wives, and his children and their wives, and all the grandchildren living together in one home. This is likely to increase the dose of airborne infection passed to members of the household and so influence severity of disease. The high case fatality from measles in West Africa is thought to result from the large family size of polygamous peoples. Children are more likely to be infected by a family member and hence to receive a larger dose of virus.

Family structure is related to many aspects of health other than communicable disease, for example to the nutrition of children and the utilization of health services.

OCCUPATION

Occupation may be related to disease frequency in at least three ways: by association with exposure to special risks and agents of disease; through selection of certain kinds of individual into certain occupations; because of an association between occupation and socioeconomic status.

Occupation and exposure to disease

Occupation may be related to special risks such as exposure to chemicals or dusts which are either ingested (e.g. organophosphates in herbicides) absorbed through the skin (e.g. silicates in bare-foot farmers in Ethiopia) or inhaled (e.g. asbestosis in miners in Zimbabwe). Trauma from a variety of physical agents is a well-known occupational hazard. Work may also bring an individual into contact with vectors or reservoirs of infectious disease: for example, cattle herders are liable to sleeping sickness and water carriers to guinea worm.

If it is suspected that a disorder is associated with a particular occupation or industrial process it is necessary for the investigator to scrutinize every phase of the job or process, for liability to the disease may attend only one small aspect of it. Even apparently simple procedures, such as tapping rubber or preparing copra, are found on analysis to involve many different activities.

Occupation and selection of workers

Some occupations select certain types of worker. The stronger, taller man may cut the sugarcane or join the army, and all such men may come from one area of the country. They will bring into the occupational group the endemic diseases of that area, perhaps schistosomiasis or kala-azar.

Occupation and socioeconomic status

In urban societies occupation is linked with socioeconomic status. Doctors, for example, are prone to obesity because their occupation usually confers on them a high standard of living.

SOCIOECONOMIC STATUS

In Europe and North America occupation is closely linked with education and standard of living. A social class classification was devised in Britain 50 years ago and is based on a grading of occupations according to their level of skill and financial rewards, and on the general status they confer in the community. In this classification there are five classes:

Social Class 1   Leading professions and business (e.g. doctor)
Social Class 2   Lesser professions and business (e.g. teacher, shopkeeper)
Social Class 3   Skilled workers, non-manual workers (e.g. clerks)
Social Class 4   Partly skilled workers (e.g. machine operators, agricultural workers)
Social Class 5   Unskilled workers (e.g. porters, labourers)

This classification defines broad categories of standards of living (income, housing, education, child-rearing practices, and attitudes towards health) and also a grading of status within the community. It has proved useful in epidemiological studies; diseases such as chronic bronchitis show marked social class differences in frequency which can be related to environmental influences such as housing and overcrowding.

In rural areas of developing countries all the people may be farmers and the only differentiation between them may be that some own tractors or use insecticides or have latrines. This differentiation is often the result of differences in educational level, which lead to differences in standards of living and hence to differences in patterns of disease. For rural populations the level of education is therefore a useful indication of socioeconomic status.

The concept of socioeconomic stratification of a society is important because often the upper social classes have low overall morbidity rates (but get the subsidized housing, special medical care, health education programmes and extra allowances), whereas the lower classes have high mortality and disability rates and should be the priority groups to receive the limited health resources in a developing country.

In analytic epidemiology an association between a disease and social class may indicate possible determinants. In this context two points must be borne in mind. Firstly, an association between a disease and social class may be secondary to an association with influences which determine social class. Endomyocardial fibrosis in Uganda is more frequent in the lowest socioeconomic group because the disease is common among Rwandan immigrants and, like immigrants in many other countries, they tend to be in the lowest socioeconomic group. The primary association of this disease appears to be with ethnic group. Secondly, diseases such as psychosis and alcoholism are common in the lower socioeconomic groups partly because psychotics and alcoholics tend to move down the social scale and end up as manual labourers or unemployed people living in the slums of cities.

Definition of socioeconomic status

In addition to educational differences, rural societies may be differentiated into landowners, tenant land-holders, settled immigrants or landless labourers. The landowners may include aristocrats, chiefs, civil servants, and educated people, as well as farmers who have been successful and have been able to buy land. Socioeconomic status may also arise from historical associations, occupational differences, descent groups, or from administrative, political or religious office.

In rural areas the epidemiologist usually has to base a classification of socioeconomic status on education, occupation or land-owning status. Other criteria which have been used are type of house, area of cultivated land, place of residence, number of cattle or pigs, mode of transport or possession of certain items such as a radio or furniture.

Different classifications will emphasize different biological aspects of socioeconomic status. Education may be reflected in hygiene practices, occupation in household income and land-owning in the availability of food.

With the movement of people to towns the differentiation into classes may become more marked, with the emergence of an élite group having incomes perhaps 10 to 20 times that of the peasant. Educational level has again often proved the most useful criterion for classifying the middle strata. Children and wives' social class should usually be taken from that of father or husband, but the frequency of some common childhood diseases may be more closely related to the educational level of the mother rather than the father.

No single socioeconomic grouping will be appropriate to urban areas in many different countries but one basis for classifying urban populations in Africa is the definition of classes by education, occupation and income.

Class 1: Highest income. Jobs requiring higher education, e.g. doctor, headmasters, company directors, senior civil servants.

Class 2: Skilled occupations requiring secondary education, e.g.

schoolteachers, technicians, nursing sisters, foremen, officers in police, army or prison service.

Class 3: Occupations requiring upper primary or lower secondary education, e.g. clerks, post office workers, auxiliary nurses, drivers, mechanics, machine operators, painters. This class may be subdivided into occupations in which suits or uniforms are worn (e.g. clerks); these jobs are usually better paid than occupations where overalls are worn (e.g. mechanics).

Class 4: Occupations requiring primary education at a lower level only, and for which suits or uniforms are usually worn, e.g. messengers, shop assistants, waiters.

Class 5: Lowest income. No education or formal training required, e.g. gardeners, labourers, street cleaners.

PLACE

Description of the variations in disease incidence between countries, or within different parts of one country, is of importance both because the information is fundamental to the planning of health services and because these variations may provide important clues to the aetiology of disease.

Mapping of the *world distribution* of diseases must usually depend on routine statistics derived from death certificates, hospital returns, notifications of infectious disease or registers of diseases such as tuberculosis and cancer. These routine data only allow crude comparisons of disease incidence between countries, for there are marked international variations in availability of medical care, diagnostic standards, and reporting of illness and death. Therefore the striking geographical variations in disease incidence shown in WHO statistical reports and similar publications must be interpreted against a background of uncertainty about the quality of the data.

The broad outlines of the world distribution of common parasitic and infectious diseases is apparent from clinical experience, for in some countries diseases such as malaria have a very high prevalence while elsewhere they are virtually absent. These international differences have been further documented by routine statistics and field surveys. Among non-infectious diseases there are many striking differences between countries. For example, recent work on cancer distributions has revealed that sub-Saharan African countries have high incidences of primary carcinoma of the oesophagus, penis and liver and low incidences of colonic and breast carcinoma in comparison with Europe and North America. The study of influences which could determine these international differences offers a method of investigating cancer aetiology.

An approximate map of disease distribution *within a country* may also be obtained from death certificates, notifications of infectious disease, and hospital and clinic returns. In developing countries certification of cause of death is not often carried out, and usually only a minority of cases of infectious disease are notified. Hospital and clinic returns give a distorted picture of disease incidence: many patients do not seek medical care; hospitals tend to be centred in towns and are less accessible to rural communities; and standards of diagnosis and reporting vary from one hospital to another. Nevertheless marked variations in disease incidence between one area to another may be revealed by hospital returns. In India returns from hospitals treating railway employees have shown that acute myocardial infarction is more common in the south than in the north. This observation has been correlated with dietary differences in the two parts of the country.

Accurate mapping of disease distribution in a developing country will usually require field surveys in which prevalence or incidence of the disease is measured in samples of the population. The investigator may record either the number of cases of active disease in the samples or the number of individuals with evidence of having had the disease at some time in the past. Evidence of previous exposure to a disease includes scars (as in yaws), disabilities (such as blindness from trachoma or muscle-wasting from polio), or elevations in blood enzyme or antibody levels (as in toxoplasmosis).

Detailed mapping of disease occurrence in one locality is an important part of the investigation and control of epidemics, as described in Chapter 9. Local maps of disease are also an integral part of many investigations of disease aetiology, even though the investigation may be based primarily on clinical or laboratory observations. No doctor's office is complete without maps, preferably mounted on soft board into which mapping pins may be inserted. Time spent in seeking out the most accurate and up-to-date maps is often well rewarded and it may be possible to obtain aerial photographs of an area. Sometimes the degree of detail on existing maps is inadequate and will need to be supplemented by the personal observations of the doctor and staff. Pins of different colours may be used to plot out cases of disease, with each colour representing an age-group or sex, or the time of onset, or the source of notification. It is surprising how patterns of disease distribution often become apparent when mapped out in this way, and study of the patterns may lead to hypotheses about the association of diseases with particular groups of people or with geographical features such as rivers, roads, or mountains.

As with age and sex there are three factors which may influence the geographical distribution of a disease.

Population density and structure

Unless a disease has a special predilection for sparsely populated areas it is likely that there will be more cases in areas of high population density. Therefore maps of disease will show clusterings of cases around towns, trading centres, and densely settled land, and may be misleading. An investigator making a local map will usually be aware of the approximate population distribution but wherever possible it is desirable to express the number of cases in each place as rates, related to the total population. To achieve greater comparability between areas these rates, whether incidences or prevalences, should be standardized for age and sex (Ch. 8). Standardization may be of particular importance in comparisons of urban and rural areas, for the age and sex distribution of urban and rural populations can be markedly different.

Levels of ascertainment

The numbers of cases of a disease recorded by a hospital and clinic may be markedly influenced by the willingness or ability of the population to seek medical treatment. Patients with leprosy, for example, are often unwilling to seek treatment. Many communities live far from hospitals or clinics and sick people are often unable to travel long distances. For a variety of reasons the ascertainment of cases of a disease by the use of existing medical records may be markedly incomplete, and even field surveys carried out in the villages may fail to achieve full ascertainment. Comparison of disease rates in areas where the levels of ascertainment differ markedly will be misleading.

Diagnostic criteria

The need for standardized observations in epidemiology is discussed in Chapter 2, and in surveys the presence or absence of a disease in an individual must be recorded in accordance with predetermined diagnostic criteria. Standardization of diagnosis enables direct comparisons to be made between the results of one survey and another. However, in routine clinical work there are often pronounced regional differences in diagnostic practice. For example, criteria for the diagnosis of early skin lesions in leprosy vary in different centres; pathologists use varying criteria for the diagnosis of early forms of cervical cancer; and technicians vary in their ability to find parasites or to culture bacteria. Apparent regional variations in disease incidence may therefore arise solely from variations in diagnostic and recording procedures. When clinical records are used for disease mapping this possible source of bias must be considered.

Interpretation of geographical distributions

If the variations in disease incidence shown on a map are not attributable to the three factors described, an explanation may be sought in terms of the distribution of determinants of the disease. Determinants of diseases which influence their geographical distribution may be grouped under three headings: characteristics of ethnic groups; the biological, physical and chemical environment; and residential environment.

Characteristics of ethnic groups

Members of an ethnic group may have a high frequency of certain genes, such as the gene for sickling, or may share certain customs, such as abstinence from alcohol, which determine high or low disease incidences within the group. In order to confirm that the geographical distribution of a disease is determined by the characteristics of an ethnic group one may look for evidence that (1) the disease occurs in all areas inhabited by the group, (2) the disease has a lower incidence in other ethnic groups inhabiting the same areas, and (3) migration of the group is followed by a rise in incidence in the new area of habitation.

The biological, physical and chemical environment

The geographical features of a place, such as climate, altitude and soil composition, determine the occurrence of a wide range of disease determinants, for example parasites, insect vectors, microorganisms, essential chemicals such as iodine, and atmospheric pollution. If the geographical distribution of a disease is determined by a particular environment then it will generally affect all ethnic groups exposed to the environment and not those outside it; migration of an ethnic group to other environments will be followed by a decline in disease incidence within the group.

Residential environment

The residential environment which a place provides may expose the inhabitants to a wide range of disease determinants. The slums of cities offer an unfavourable environment which results from the interplay of patterns of occupation, social relationship, diet, availability of medical services, and influences in the biological, physical and chemical environment. In comparison a new industrial town in Sierra Leone has been shown to have a favourable residential environment; the general health of its residents is better than that of the population in the surrounding villages.

TIME

Changes in disease frequency with time are represented by histograms or frequency polygons (Ch. 8) in which the frequency of the disease is plotted on the vertical axis and time, on the appropriate scale, on the horizontal axis. Usually disease frequency is related to time of onset of the disease (if there are accurate data on this), rather than time of diagnosis, admission to hospital or death. This distinction of time of onset from time of events in the subsequent course of the disease may be unimportant in the analysis of a cholera epidemic, where the progress and outcome of the disease are swift, but for a chronic disease such trachoma the pattern of frequency of diagnosis with time will be a distorted reflection of the pattern of frequency of onset with time, since long intervals may separate onset and diagnosis. Changes in disease frequency may be considered under three headings, according to the time scale involved — epidemics, cyclic changes and secular changes.

Epidemics

In current usage the word 'epidemic' refers to any marked upward fluctuation in disease incidence or prevalence. The sharp increase in traffic accident deaths in Africa during the past few years is as much an epidemic as the sudden outbreaks of meningococcal meningitis which sweep across West Africa. However, knowledge of the patterns of epidemic fluctuations has been mainly derived from

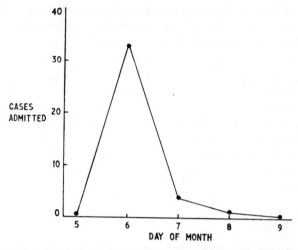

Fig. 5.4   Cases of 'barley-poisoning' admitted to hospital in Singapore.

study of epidemics of infectious disease spread over a few weeks or months.

Figure 5.4 shows the pattern of a *point-source epidemic* in which more or less simultaneous exposure of many susceptible individuals to a source of pathogenic organisms or chemicals results in an explosive increase in the number of cases of the disease over a short period. An epidemic of poisoning with an insecticide called para-

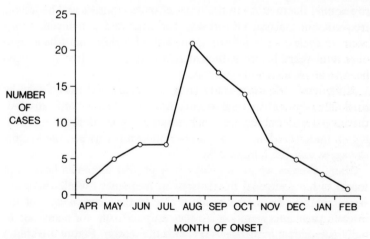

Fig. 5.5   Number of cases of poliomyelitis with residual paralysis, by month of onset, in the Kolda Region of Senegal, from 1986–1987. Source: Centers of Disease Control, Atlanta.

thion occurred in Singapore as a result of consumption of contaminated barley. On the first day of the epidemic there·were 33 cases (6 deaths). Vigorous public health measures prevented further consumption of the barley and there were no further cases after 3 days. In contrast, Figure 5.5 shows the pattern of a *contagious disease epidemic* in which an organism is propagated in the community by passage from person to person, so that the initial rise in the number of cases is less abrupt than in point-source epidemics. The figure shows the numbers of confirmed cases of poliomyelitis each month in Kolda Region, Senegal, during 1986–1987. The peak number of admissions occurred 5 months after the apparent onset of the epidemic.

Cyclic changes

Some diseases are observed to undergo cyclical changes in frequency during the course of days, weeks, months, seasons or years. The onset of hayfever tends to occur at certain times of the day, in relation to the diurnal rhythm of household activities such as sweeping the house and going to the fields. Attendance at gonorrhoea clinics has been found to show a weekly peak on Tuesdays and Wednesdays, as a result of peak transmission rates over the weekend. In some places the practice of paying salaried employees on the last day of each month leads to an increase in head injuries on the first day of the month. Seasonal variations in rainfall lead to seasonal fluctuations in the number of mosquitoes and hence the frequency of malaria. Outbreaks of measles and poliomyelitis may occur in cycles, since following one outbreak there must be a lapse of several years before sufficient non-immune children have been born to allow a second outbreak.

Nutritional deficiency states such as pellagra and rickets may be markedly seasonal in their occurrence. For vector-borne diseases the investigation of any seasonal variations in incidence is essential for an understanding of the inter-relationship between the vector, the agent and the human host.

Many diseases whose aetiology is at present unknown have been found to have seasonal fluctuations in frequency. While these observations may seem to provide a clue to the determinants of the disease, their interpretation is necessarily difficult, for many potentially pathogenic influences vary with the season. Figure 5.6 shows the pattern of meningococcal disease in Zaria, Nigeria. It is not known whether the increase in numbers of cases in the middle of

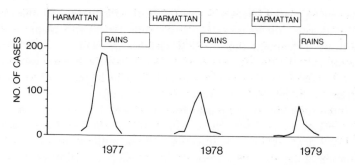

Fig. 5.6 Numbers of cases of meningococcal disease admitted to a hospital in Zaria, Nigeria each month during 3 years. Periods of rain and the Harmattan wind are also shown.

the year is due to the low humidity, the Harmattan wind, or seasonal changes in people's behaviour. Not only do the seasons influence the animal and plant environment, with changes in the breeding of vectors and hosts of disease, but there are seasonal changes in many aspects of human behaviour, such as occupation, diet and recreation. However, cyclic changes in incidence sometimes provide crucial evidence about aetiology. Pork has been implicated as the vector of the pig-bel syndrome (necrotizing jejunitis) in New Guinea because its cyclic peaks of incidence coincide with cyclic pig-feasting practices. For other diseases the demonstration of cyclic variations in frequency is helpful only in so far as hypotheses about determinants may be untenable unless the determinants show corresponding cyclic variations.

Secular changes

Changes in disease incidence over periods of many years are referred to as secular changes. The past hundred years have seen dramatic movements of peoples from one country to another, and many once-isolated countries are now exposed to the constant passage of visitors. Accompanying this new freedom of travel has been the dissemination of infectious diseases so that cholera, for example, is now widespread in countries where it was previously unknown. It may be predicted that economic development, involving as it does major changes in the way of life of a people, will bring with it marked changes in disease patterns during the next decades. The rapid urbanization and industrialization of developing countries may bring marked secular increases in the incidence of ischaemic heart disease, diabetes, gallstones, mental illness and many other diseases. Documentation of these changes in incidence will be of importance for the organization of health care, and may also give a new insight into the aetiology of diseases which comprise the main threat to the health of industrialized communities.

Interesting and important as they are, long-term changes in disease incidence are difficult to demonstrate. The usual sources of data are death certificates, infectious disease notifications and sometimes hospital and clinic records. In developing countries, where the first two sources may be unavailable, knowledge of secular changes may depend on observations made at a few hospitals whose records go back many years. Where changes in incidence have been dramatic, such as the disappearance of malaria from Mauritius following eradication programmes, general clinical experience may indicate them, but most changes will not be revealed by such a relatively insensitive method of detection.

When interpreting changes in disease frequency over periods of many years it is necessary to consider first the same three factors as have been considered for age, sex and place.

Population density and structure

Changes in population size will alter the number of cases of a disease. The recent rapid increase in the population of many developing countries has led to an increasing number of patients seeking medical care without necessarily any alteration of incidence. Changes in the age/sex structure of a population may also lead to changes in the numbers of cases. It may be predicted that increasing life expectancy in developing countries will lead to increasing numbers of patients with diseases such as osteoarthritis and cancer.

Levels of ascertainment

The level of ascertainment of a disease like leprosy may vary markedly in one area at different times, in accordance with changes in case-finding procedures or local attitudes to the disease. Such changes may give rise to a false impression of a secular change in incidence.

Diagnostic criteria

Changes in criteria for the diagnosis of a disease may result in an apparent change in its incidence. Diseases such as diabetes, hypertension, and anaemia pose special problems in epidemiology because their diagnosis depends on measurements which are continuously distributed in the population, and 'normal' merges imperceptibly into 'abnormal' (Fig. 3.1).

Interpretation of secular changes

When considering the reasons underlying variations in disease incidence over long periods of time it is difficult to discount the possible influences of variations in population density and structure, ascertainment or diagnosis. Whereas with geographical variations the effect of these influences is accessible to current inquiry, interpretation of secular changes depends upon inferences about observations made many years ago. Nevertheless the reality of secular changes can sometimes be established with reasonable certainty. There seems little doubt that the sharp increase in numbers of reported lung cancer deaths in the UK during the past 50 years resulted from a real increase in lung cancer incidence. Discussions of this point have provided an instructive example of the methodology of demonstrating secular changes.

The possible determinants of secular variation are similar to those of geographical variation, described in the preceding section, namely characteristics of ethnic groups, the biological, physical and chemical environment, and the residential environment.

MOVEMENT

Disease frequency can vary with place or with time. Sometimes it varies simultaneously with place and time, that is with movement. Two kinds of movement are of epidemiological importance. Firstly people may *migrate* from one area to another, taking diseases with them, removing themselves from exposure to diseases in the area they leave, or exposing themselves to new diseases in their area of settlement. Secondly diseases may move through static populations leaving *clusters* of affected persons in their path.

Migrants

The spread of infectious diseases through the movement of peoples has been a major force in world history. In 1348 merchants fleeing from the Crimea brought plague to Italy and thence to England, where for 300 years recurrent epidemics of the 'Black Death' destroyed large sections of the population. In the 19th century cholera spread out from India and since then travellers have disseminated it over a wide area of the world. Throughout the world refugees, pilgrims, travellers, nomads, armies, schoolchildren, traders, migrant labourers, prostitutes move from one place to another, taking with them their own patterns of disease, acquiring new diseases, and disseminating their own diseases to others.

Nomadic peoples pose especial problems in preventive medicine. For example, malaria eradication in Somalia is greatly hindered by the movements of nomadic peoples, who disperse over wide areas of the country to graze their cattle, and may even cross into Kenya and Ethiopia.

In descriptive studies the migrants in a population need to be distinguished from the settled peoples, since their disease patterns may differ. In Brazil a new disease 'the haemorrhagic syndrome of Altamira' was described among immigrants, who moved into the Altamira area as part of a government scheme to colonize the forests along the new Transamazon Highway. The illness was characterized by cutaneous and mucosal haemorrhages associated with thrombocytopenia, and did not occur among the local people. In their new settlements the immigrants were greatly troubled by the bites of Simulium flies during the rainy season. The local people mostly lived in the city where simulidae are fewer. The restriction of the disease to immigrants was one of the epidemiological and serological observations which led to the hypothesis that the disease is a hypersensitivity phenomenon or response to a toxin associated with intense Simulium biting.

In analytic studies migrants are of special interest in two circumstances. First, when a group of people moves from an area where a disease is absent, or has a low incidence, into an area of high incidence their experience of the disease may be compared with that of the local population in the high-incidence area. The migrant group may bring with it a different pattern of immunity to the disease and through differing customs in such things as diet and housing may have a different exposure to harmful influences in the new environment. Observation of differing disease frequencies in immigrant and native groups may therefore be related to hypotheses about disease causation. Migration of Polynesian communities to New Zealand is accompanied by a sharp rise in the incidence of hypertension, diabetes and gout. Study of the occurrence of these three diseases in the migrants offers a possible way of identifying their environmental causes.

Secondly, when a group of people moves from an area of high incidence of a disease into an area where the disease has a low incidence or is absent, observation of the change in incidence may be informative. The migrating group takes with it disease determinants related to its genetic structure or to certain of its fixed customs, such as circumcision of the male infant, but it is freed from exposure to harmful influences in the environment it is leaving. Observation of the rate of decline in disease incidence in the migrants may be pertinent to determination of the latent period between exposure to an environmental influence and appearance of the disease. A group of 2500 Rwandan refugees in Uganda, of whom some 300 had suffered from mycobacterial skin ulcers during a 3-year period, were moved to a new settlement outside the area where the disease occurs. After 8 weeks the incidence of the disease fell sharply and after 13 weeks no further cases occurred. Thus the latent period of the disease was revealed as being between 8 and 13 weeks.

Observation of disease incidence in migrant groups has been the basis of a number of studies of coronary artery disease and cancer, and these studies have afforded tantalizing glimpses of possible environmental determinants. The interpretation of such studies is liable to certain difficulties. Emigrants may be unrepresentative of the population they leave and their disease experience before migration may not be accurately described by reference to the population as a whole. Migration itself subjects people to unusual stresses, and the thousands of Irish emigrants who contracted and died of typhus during the journey to Canada are a testimony to this. It had been found that among Norwegian immigrants into the USA there is a higher incidence of psychosis than in Norway. Although this may point to influences in the environment of the USA which lead to psychotic illness, it may also be a result of selective emigration from Norway of less stable persons, more liable to mental illness, or of the unusual stresses imposed on immigrants during their adjustment to a foreign culture.

Clustering

An epidemic of a new disease, called o'nyong nyong fever, occurred in East Africa. It was estimated that at least a million people were affected. When the dates of highest incidence of the disease in each affected area were plotted on a map it was obvious that cases occurring in any one area tended to occur at around the same time.

This phenomenon is known as time-space clustering, and in the o'nyong nyong epidemic it was interpreted as being the result of spread of the causative virus from one community to another.

Inspection of the map of cases of o'nyong nyong was sufficient to detect clustering. However, for other diseases the clustering is not evident from simple inspection of maps showing the date of occurrence of each case, and elaborate statistical techniques are required. These techniques detect the extent to which groups of cases occurring close together geographically also tend to occur close together in time, and determine whether the degree of clustering demonstrated is greater than that which might be expected to occur by chance. Great interest has been aroused by the demonstration that, using these techniques, it is possible to demonstrate clustering in leukaemia and lymphomas. One possible inference from this is that one of the determinants of these diseases may be an infectious agent. However, although clustering may be caused by movement of a micro-organism through a community, it may also result from movement of many other kinds. Heroin addiction may show clustering, as knowledge of the drug and its abuse spreads in a community. Movements of populations and diagnostic fashions may also result in clusters of cases.

6. Records

Recording of data is an essential part of any epidemiological survey and the ease and accuracy with which this is done depend partly on the design of the record form. A carefully designed form facilitates not only the collection of data, but also its storage and analysis.

There should usually be separate records for each unit being studied, for example a person, a household, or an X-ray. Wherever possible a serial number should be incorporated in each record so that later on missing ones can be identified.

Two points about data collection deserve emphasis. First it is the fieldworker who supplies the crude data; his training, accuracy of observation, and precision of recording are of the utmost importance. Secondly the recording of data must be carefully supervised and checked for accuracy during the course of the survey.

FIELD SURVEY RECORDS

In a survey it is seldom possible to use a record form identical to one used elsewhere. Although there are a number of standardized record forms available, such as those for cardiovascular studies published by the WHO, they usually require modification to meet the particular language and other cultural characteristics of an area. Sometimes forms which an investigator has used elsewhere can be used again with a few additions and erasures, and in order to avoid having the forms reprinted, it may be possible merely to have a rubber-stamp made of the new items and to stamp them on to each form.

Record forms will need to be of thick paper or card in order to withstand repeated handling. If finances allow, a clear plastic wallet for each form will prolong its life. The size of the forms is partly dictated by the means of storage, and may range from small cards stored in drawer-files to foolscap ones stored in box or envelope files.

Detailed instructions on the use of record forms should be given in an instruction sheet. Reminders may be included on the forms themselves, including practical hints such as the use of pencils rather than pens in wet weather, when ink will run on the paper.

Personal identity

A record card for an individual must usually include age, sex, address, and personal identity or name. There are several reasons for requiring this last item although it is not used in the analysis. Some surveys require repeated observations on the same individual, for example, height, antibody titres, or serum biochemistry, and these observations must be linked together. In other surveys the investigator is under an ethical obligation to locate individuals for treatment of conditions, such as malaria parasitaemia, which are only determined when laboratory tests have been completed. Sometimes personal identification is required to prevent spread of a communicable disease or to trace contacts.

In some countries, such as Malaysia, each individual has a national identity card with a unique number. In other countries individuals' names do not change and, combined with age and address, can be readily used for identification. However, in many developing countries names and addresses change frequently, and age is seldom accurate. Continued identification of an individual may be difficult unless such items as birthplace, father's name, clan, tribe, and perhaps even fingerprints and photograph are included.

A unique identification number is helpful in linking different forms made out for the same person. It is especially important when analysis is to be made by computer. It is helpful if this unique number has some meaning. For example, a recent study recording vaccinations on children used a two-letter code for the place where the child was immunized, up to four digits for the order in which the child came for registration and two digits for the year of registration. So child number BM/134/88 is the 134th child to register for vaccination at Brikama in 1988. In studies of whole populations involving a census the identification number can include the address. S19 3 4 is the fourth child household 3 of the 19th compound of the village Si-Kunda.

The number of items on a form

When designing records it is tempting to include a number of questions and observations which, although not directly related to the main purpose of the study, may prove useful later. For example, having drawn up a record sheet to determine the prevalence of tuberculous infection by tuberculin testing, the doctor may be inclined to add a series of questions and observations on nutrition, income and education, because it is possible that these influences may be related to the pattern of tuberculous infection and may show interesting associations when analysed.

Even patients in hospital are likely to become unco-operative if subjected to lengthy interrogation and examination. In the field a person who is hurrying, or anxious about work, or bored, may either go away without completing the procedure or give hasty, inaccurate replies. Moreover a lengthy form with scores of questions may be subtly attenuated by the field workers when they see that it is taking too much time. Therefore extension of a record form to include extra questions and observations may jeopardize the accuracy of the most vital information. Generally a survey form should be restricted to as few items as is compatible with answering the specific questions for which it was designed.

The sequence of items on a form

The ease and accuracy with which information is obtained may depend on the sequence in which an interview and examination are carried out. It is usual to put a person at ease by first asking simple questions about name and address. Similarly during examination it is best to do reassuring things like weighing before items such as examination of the abdomen or blood sampling. With children the sequence of examination may be especially important, as once a child is frightened co-operation of both child and parents is lost. The sequence of items on a form should also be related to the 'line of flow' of the people being interviewed and examined (see Ch. 7), so that all the results of laboratory examinations, for example, are usually grouped together at the end of the form.

The layout of a form

If the results are to be analysed by hand careful layout of the form will allow any particular item of information to be readily identified

Filaria survey form F1

Serial no.

Date ⬚⬚⬚⬚⬚⬚

Name . . . .

Head of household . . . .

Survey number   ⬚⬚⬚⬚⬚

Village . . . .

Age (in years)   ⬚⬚

Enter Y for yes, N for no.

Sex	Male . . . . □	
	Female . . . . □	
Marital status	Married . . . . □	
	Single . . . . □	
	Divorced . . . . □	
	Separated . . . . □	
	Widowed . . . . □	
Number of people in household	1	□
	2	□
	3	□
	4	□
	5–9	□
	10–14	□
	15 and over	□

Fieldworker No.   ⬚⬚

Fig. 6.1 A simple survey record.

as each sheet is turned up. It may be helpful to use different coloured cards for different age/sex groups to enable rapid sorting.
Alternatively one corner of the forms of a certain group, such as
all children, may be cut off so that these forms can be swiftly separated from the others. The correct amount of space should be allowed for each item: often too little space is allowed and assistants
with large writing have difficulty. Layout should allow for rapid
sorting. Figure 6.1 shows an example of a simple form. It may be
noted that although this form elicits only the simplest information
the interviewers would nevertheless require careful preliminary instruction and supervision. The terms used to describe 'marital
status' must be defined; and it should be made clear whether the

'number of people in household' includes or excludes the respondent, and whether occupancy of households is defined by where people habitually sleep, or eat, or by some other criteria.

If the information from a form is to be entered into a computer, the layout is also crucial. Errors in data entry increase with the size and complexity of the form. All forms should be entered twice, compared, or 'verified', and errors corrected. This will be a tedious and time-consuming operation if the number of errors is large. Modern computer programs handle letters just as well as numbers, so there is no need to code yes and no as 1 and 2 respectively; Y and N are just as good and reduce confusion and coding errors. This is also preferable to ticking boxes, as a blank box may represent an omission, whereas N is a clear negative.

Finally it is wise always to record the identity of the fieldworker completing the form. This allows problems to be discussed with the individual concerned, forms from a particular fieldworker, later found to be unreliable, to be separated and encourages care in form-filling.

Coded forms

The analysis of a survey is facilitated if the data are coded at the time of collection. The question 'how often do you go fishing?' may elicit replies ranging from 'every day' to 'never'. If these replies are recorded using the respondent's own words it will be necessary to categorize and group them at the time of analysis. Time is saved if this is done at the time of interview and the replies are recorded as, for example, one of four alternatives: (1) daily, (2) weekly, (3) monthly or (4) never. This is *pre-coding*.

If there are more than about a thousand records analysis becomes difficult unless computer processing is used. This will necessitate transfer of the data from the forms into the computer (described in a later section of this chapter). Pre-coding is needed as it may prove difficult to code information recorded in free form. For example, the type of roof on the respondent's home may be recorded as 'permanent' when the investigator wishes to categorize replies into 'galvanized iron' or 'asbestos cement.' Pre-coding requires prior knowledge of the categories of answer that will be obtained and therefore pilot or trial surveys may be necessary.

The nature of the information determines to a large extent the degree of detail that can be coded. With numerical data it is necessary to decide on the degree of accuracy required, and whether the data are to be grouped. (The WHO has published a number of codes, such as the International Classification of Disease, which covers causes of mortality and morbidity and is repeatedly revised to meet statistical and medical needs.)

When data on forms are to be entered into a computer it is advisable to ask the data entry clerks to comment on the form when it is first drafted. They may request a particular kind of layout to enable rapid processing. For large studies special data entry programs can be written which produce a picture of the form on the visual display unit. This simplifies data entry.

The record shown in Figure 6.1 could be pre-coded as shown in Figure 6.2. This has been completed, with X in the relevant boxes, for a single man of 20–24 years who lives in Bulamu village in a household comprising three persons. An alternative to using an X is to draw a circle round the number in the relevant box. This has an advantage in that the number is not obscured; but if carelessly drawn the circle may overlap two boxes so that it is unclear as to which is the correct one.

INTERVIEW OR QUESTIONNAIRE FORMS

The design of interview forms requires careful thought. For the epidemiologist, it is the equivalent to the basic scientist's laboratory method. Sometimes it is necessary to specify the exact wording of each question in advance to achieve uniformity in the replies elicited by different workers (i.e. to minimize between-observer variation as described in Ch. 2). A woman may give different accounts of her family according to whether she is asked 'how many children have you?' 'how many children have you had?' or 'how many children are there in your family?' If these questions are being asked in a language different from the investigator's there may be further pitfalls. It is advisable to get several workers to translate the questions into the local language and then to have them translated back into the investigator's language to see if the intent of the questions has been preserved. In certain cultures there are acceptable and unacceptable ways of phrasing questions about topics such as death and disorders of women. In one part of Papua direct questions about menstruation are considered offensive and a more delicate approach is necessary; the woman should be asked whether she has recently 'seen the moon'.

If the questions asked are such that people may have difficulty in answering them accurately, or will be unwilling to do so, it may

Filaria survey form F1

Serial No. 693

Date | 2 | 9 | 0 | 6 | 8 | 6 |

Name: *James Musoke*

Head of household: *Charles Nakibinge*

Column				
1–4	Survey number	0	8	5	3

INDICATE CORRECT BOX WITH X

Column						
5	Village	Bulamu [X]	Kasangati 2	Wampewo 3	Other* 4	
		*specify:				

Column							
6	Age (in years)	0–4 1	5–9 2	10–14 3	15–19 4	20–24 [X] 5	25+ 6
7	Sex	M [X]	F 2				
8	Marital status	Married 1	Single [X] 2	Divorced 3	Separated 4	Widowed 5	
9	Number of people in household	1	2	3 [X]	4	5	6	7
		1	2	3	4	5–9	10–14	15+

Fig. 6.2 A pre-coded survey record.

be better to allow the interviewer to vary the form of the questions according to the persons being interviewed. In some parts of East Africa people are unwilling to disclose the fact that they are obtaining water from nearby swamps rather than walking further to the nearest borehole. During interviews under these circumstances it has been found useful to begin with general questions about the availability of water for washing, bathing and drinking at different seasons, and then to lead on to specific questions about the use of swamps. Often it is satisfactory to specify an initial question and then indicate how the interviewer should probe further depending on the answers received.

In order to avoid exposing all participants in a survey to a lengthy interview, it may be advisable to devise two questionnaires, one short and the other long. The short one comprises the essential questions and is given to all persons interviewed. The long one has additional questions and is administered to a sample of the participants. Sometimes a long questionnaire may be required for one category of person, such as women in the child-bearing age.

In *attitude surveys* it is usual to arrange the questions so that the respondent replies along a scale of agreement varying from complete agreement through indifference to complete disagreement. The attitudes to be tested should be put either from a negative or positive point of view at random, for example 'it is harmful for a woman to eat eggs', or 'it is beneficial for a woman to eat eggs'. Double-barrelled statements should be avoided, for example 'it is harmful for a woman to eat eggs and she should be divorced if she does so'. A person may agree with the first attitude but disagree with the second, and will be confused as to overall response.

Attitude questionnaires are difficult to construct, and it may be advisable for the investigator to consult one of the many books written on the subject (such as Abramson's book on survey methods; see Suggested Further Reading, p. 169) or to obtain expert guidance from a social psychologist familiar with the particular culture.

In some circumstances *postal questionnaires* may be used, with obvious saving in time and money. For example, in order to obtain a crude estimate of the frequency of poliomyelitis in a district of Ghana a postal questionnaire was sent to the head teachers of 88 schools. The questionnaire asked them to list lame children in their school or village. The success of this method led to the suggestion that it should be more widely used as a method of assessing the frequency of polio and the impact of immunization. However low literacy rates and poor postal services preclude the use of self-administered questionnaires in many countries.

CLINIC RECORDS

On occasions an investigator may want clinic staff to obtain information for him, and to do this will have to design an additional record to be completed for certain types of patient. However, the request to record additional data is often not met, because clinic staff tend to be too busy to take on additional paper-work. In these circumstances the investigator can employ a full-time clerk to complete the forms or may have to limit his requirements to data obtainable from the standard clinic records. Alternatively the clinic staff may be asked to obtain sufficient identification data, such as name, age, and address, to enable the investigator to follow up the patients at a later date; or the staff may give suitable patients an appointment to return to the clinic at a time when the investigator and his team are present.

SPECIAL TYPES OF RECORD

Computer records

With the falling price of personal computers and their widespread accessibility most investigators will use them to analyse their data, even in small studies. However, there are specific problems of computer usage in the tropics.

A computer needs to be kept at a reasonable ambient temperature and in many places will require an air-conditioned room for at least part of the year. The temperature in the room will need to be within the range 12–18°C. Dust, which will jam disk drives, can be controlled by ensuring that the computer is kept as far from the outside environment as possible, with a number of intervening doors. If there are frequent interruptions to the power supply, or large fluctuations in current, an uninterruptible power supply and a voltage stabilizer will be needed. These may be more expensive than the computer itself.

It is preferable to select a computer whose manufacturers have a maintenance agent in the country, and which other people in the country already have or will have. This allows the sharing of spare parts and experience.

The maintenance of a back-up copy of data is essential lest the primary data be damaged. It will need to be up-dated at regular intervals, perhaps weekly, and may be stored on floppy disks. These disks can be corrupted when transported by sea freight, and should therefore be imported by air. It is advisable to store them under the same conditions as the main computer. An additional back-up copy should be stored at a different site, perhaps the investigator's home, in case the computer building is destroyed by fire or in some other way.

A computer should preferably have a hard disk. These are more reliable than floppy disks under tropical conditions. They should have the facility for transferring data on to floppy disks, which are needed to send data to other people or transfer them on to a mainframe computer. If the latter is planned the microcomputer must be compatible with the mainframe both in terms of floppy disks and software.

The computer must be able to support the software, that is ready-made programs, needed for the study. Relational databases are useful for epidemiological work. They store different aspects of the overall data in different files and simplify their manipulation. Obviously, an understanding of what the computer is doing with the data is essential to proper analysis.

Computer records can be used to improve the management of a study. In a study of morbidity from malaria the basic census data on a group of 389 children formed the core of the data. During the rainy season weekly questionnaires were administered to the children's mothers. These data were entered at the end of the week and checked for consistency and logic by a specially written computer program. Inappropriately answered and unanswered questions were isolated. These were discussed with the fieldworker responsible before the next weekly round of questionnaires, and inconsistencies were corrected while the interview was fresh in the fieldworker's mind. In a similar way the identification data of all children in a rotavirus vaccine trial were entered on a computer at entry to the study. This allowed weekly lists of children due for vaccination to be generated and used by fieldworkers in home-visiting. This improved compliance with the intended vaccination schedule. Similar methodologies have been developed for continuous demographic monitoring of populations.

Recently, handheld computers have been developed into which interviews can be directly entered in the field by the interviewer. These can check the responses on the spot for consistency and logic. They have the added advantage of eliminating data entry, as the memory chip can be removed from them and placed in a microcomputer. These sophisticated methods are under trial at present. However, there must be reservations about their effect on response rates in rural areas.

Tape-recorders

During fieldwork tape-recordings of interviews may prove useful.

A small transistorized cassette model with built-in microphone is the most suitable for this purpose, since the person interviewed feels less self-conscious than if asked to speak directly into a microphone. Tape-recordings are helpful in overcoming language difficulties, since additional opinions can be sought on the exact meaning of words and phrases used in an interview. A tape-recorder may also be useful for recording complex directions for finding a house or village. As a fieldworker drives along he can describe in sequence the landmarks he is passing so that another worker can later use the tape as directions for follow-up visits. An alternative is to teach drivers how to make maps. If they accompany subjects home from a clinic they can then accurately locate the home for follow-up visits.

Diaries, logbooks and registers

A useful form of survey record is the daily diary describing the place, the numbers of people seen, and the problems encountered. Similarly records of travel can be noted in a logbook. When writing these informal records the investigator must bear in mind that if the notes are too brief and cryptic they may be incomprehensible when he refers to them, perhaps 6 months or a year later.

Registers are unsatisfactory records as it is time-consuming to extract information from them unless the number of items is small. However, it is often useful to record in a register the names, addresses, serial numbers and perhaps other details of all persons in a survey. The register then serves as an index enabling people to be traced, or missing documents to be found.

Photographs

Photographic records of individuals or houses facilitate their identification at a later date. Sequential changes, such as increase in size of a leprosy lesion or a seasonal change in agricultural practice, are also conveniently documented by photographs.

Other records

Certain investigations constitute records in themselves, for example X-rays, electrocardiographs or electrophoretic strips. They should be filed with identification numbers that link them with records of interviews or examination.

RECORD LINKAGE

Sometimes several records, from different sources, are compiled for each individual in a survey. For example, a mother's antenatal record may be separate from her delivery and postnatal record, or patients may have a clinical record, compiled by medical staff, and a social record compiled by other workers. An essential preliminary to the analysis of this kind of data is the linkage of all records related to a single individual. The problems of record linkage have received considerable attention in industrialized countries where the computer's capacity for rapid data-processing has been used to link large series of records. In Birmingham, UK, for example, the obstetric records of 50 000 children have been linked to the records of their school performance at the age of 11 years. This has enabled analysis of the association between obstetric complications and impaired intellectual development.

Record linkage demands that each individual has unique identification which occurs on all records relating to him or her, and that the linked records for each individual must be stored in a way that allows their rapid retrieval for the addition of new information. Record linkage is considered further during discussion of preventive trials (Ch. 10).

TRANSPORT AND STORAGE OF RECORDS

At the end of a survey each record may represent a large expenditure, perhaps £50 or more, and as such is valuable and often irreplaceable. It is therefore advisable to duplicate records so that a complete set is retained if the originals have to be transported or are otherwise exposed to loss. This is most conveniently done by photocopying each record. Special care must be taken in tropical areas to protect records against the effects of climate and insect damage. In large long-term studies it may be necessary to have an air-conditioned store. Efficient transport and storage of records require not only their protection from loss but also preservation of the confidential nature of the information they contain.

7. Fieldwork techniques

Chapter 1 gives an outline of the sequence of decisions and actions which must be taken by an investigator responsible for the administration of an epidemiological survey. The sequence is considered under four phases: planning; organization; execution; evaluation and feedback (see Ch. 11). Each of these phases demands consideration of basic problems such as sample selection, or choice of controls, which are described in other chapters of this book. In addition there are a large number of practical considerations to be taken into account. Although many of them may seem trivial or obvious their neglect may cause failure of the survey. At the outset of any survey it is wise to make an informal visit to the area to see whether the local people recognize the need for the survey, and will support it.

PLANNING

Formalities before commencing fieldwork

National formalities

Before field research can be undertaken in many developing countries it is necessary to obtain permission from the Ministry of Health, or from a National Research Council which co-ordinates and selects research priorities. Applications for permission to conduct research must be precise as to the objectives and the ultimate use and value of the results which may be obtained. They should indicate the observations to be made, the methods to be employed, e.g. questionnaires or blood sampling, the population to be studied, the source and allocation of funds and the experience and qualifications of the investigators. Even if there are no formalities involving research or ethical committees, a scientific investigation always requires careful consideration of its value and ethics. Inexperienced research workers tend to spend insufficient time in specifying their objectives and methods at the outset of an investigation.

Local formalities

In addition to national formalities there are usually local formal channels of approach which vary with the particular culture or society. In some countries the line of authority extends through a chain of county, parish and village chiefs whose permission must be sought in order of rank.

Preliminary appraisal of the area

When planning a survey the choice of population and the selection of a sample from it are among the first considerations, and require some preliminary knowledge of the demography and residential pattern of the people. A list of villages, a map of a town, or a list of taxpayers is of value if accompanied by data on where people live and who they are in terms of age, sex and ethnic group. In one district of Uganda the homes are scattered over the hills and there is a large immigrant population. In another district the residences of the population are mainly confined to a strip of land near to permanent water sources: the people live in large extended family units and at certain times of the year the men are absent herding cattle. In many countries surveys are made easier by the existence of compact villages.

The demographic information necessary for planning must be obtained well in advance. Sometimes it can be found in offices, but often it is only obtained by travelling and visiting the area to be surveyed. Driving through a valley, sitting in a bar talking to the local people, or spending a few days in the local administrative centre will not be wasted time.

Sometimes it is necessary to map and take a census of an area in order to determine the total population and have a framework for selecting a sample. Aerial photographs and large-scale maps can often be obtained from government survey offices and will form the basis for more detailed mapping on foot. Where authority is highly structured a list of local chiefs or chairmen may form an adequate framework from which to select a population sample.

Preliminary inspection of an area by vehicle or on foot, and subsequent census-taking with all the questioning that it entails, is often made difficult by the population's fears — perhaps that it is being done to find tax defaulters. In some localities people dislike having their children counted as this 'tempts fate to reduce the number'. The field staff have to be sensitive to local attitudes so that their preliminary work encourages collaboration with the survey.

Cultural influences must be considered in all phases of a field survey, and the investigator must learn about the people in the area. Actual pre-survey travel in the area is important; discussion with old people is often informative; and anthropological, sociological, economic and geographical books and papers will extend the investigator's knowledge.

Timing of a survey

The duration of the rainy season and the availability of transport are two important things to consider in the timing of a survey.

It is also important to carry out a survey at a time when the population is able to participate. Seasonal activities may take all the women away to the fields, or religious holidays may prevent any work being done at all. Coincidence of a survey with tax-collecting can be a disaster. In rural areas agricultural and pastoral activities should be studied, as on the one hand it may be difficult for people to spare time at busy periods such as harvesting or planting, whereas on the other hand activities such as a cotton sale, for which people gather together, may make a survey easier. Seasonal activities may make the population resident in a village unrepresentative of the population as a whole: perhaps at one time of the year the men go away to graze their cattle and at another time the children go to scare birds from the crops.

ORGANIZATION

Community collaboration

The people

A good relationship between the survey team and the population being surveyed is essential if there is to be the required response and coverage. People will participate if they want and support the investigation and have no unjustified fears about it. Therefore they must be adequately informed about it, perhaps at an initial community meeting. This information must lead to motivation to participate. Prompt treatment of illness and easy referral to hospital, a feeling of benefiting the community or science in general may all play a part in ensuring a good relationship. People should be assured that treatment will be arranged, usually through the existing health services, or provided on the spot for common conditions such as scabies, impetigo, conjunctivitis, minor wounds or tinea. In general health surveys, when laboratory tests are being done, malaria, hookworm and ascariasis may also be treated. The treatment of ascariasis gives especially dramatic results which are usually much appreciated.

In addition to treating common disease conditions found in individual patients the investigator may wish to broaden his survey so that it brings more public health benefit to the population. Immunization and health education can thus be added to a survey primarily intended to find the distribution of haemoglobin types. It is suggested that 'no survey without service' should be adopted as a slogan for all epidemiological studies. Care must be taken that such service is in agreement with government policy and is given with the approval of the local health authorities.

If complicated procedures which are unfamiliar to the population are being done, for example electrocardiogram recording, then it is necessary to explain them and also to describe the possible benefits they may confer. Investigations and treatment that are unpleasant or cause occasional severe side-effects should be avoided if possible; thus every effort should be made to use capillary rather than venous blood samples, and drugs such as chloroquine should be given by mouth rather than by injection.

When communicating with local people with whose culture he is not closely familiar the investigator must beware of the 'fallacy of the empty pot'. The basis of the fallacy is the idea that people are like empty pots into which new information may be poured. In fact they are not empty and have their own ideas which will influence their perception and reception of the investigator's message. Before a survey it is therefore wise to study people's recognition of the condition being investigated, their ideas of causation, and what they think and feel about it. Many endemic diseases are so common that people regard them as a variation of normal. For instance among some peoples a large hydrocele from filarial infection is regarded as usual, and other peoples regard the haematuria of bilharzia in young boys as a normal developmental stage. In areas of endemic onchocerciasis the appearance of the skin is so universal that it does not arouse comment. Traditional ideas of causation and spread of such diseases seldom invoke insect vectors or faecal contamination.

If people have no knowledge of parasites but believe an illness to be due to a 'bewitchment', or the 'evil eye', or that it is a penalty for some wrong behaviour, then it will need special effort to convince them at a single meeting of the need for a stool or urine specimen to detect parasites. These early discussions can form the basis for an on-going dialogue with the community. This gives opportunities for discussion of difficulties and problems with the study.

Sampling procedures used in the selection of particular individuals or households to be investigated often create suspicion. People may ask 'why was I chosen and not my neighbour?' Cluster sampling will overcome this problem, and explanation of the rationale of sampling is usually accepted. Local analogies can be used, based on everyday sampling in market purchasing, for example examination of a few potatoes from different parts of a sack to determine the quality of the whole sackful.

The leaders

Important people, and religious and unofficial leaders of the community, must be specially briefed about a survey because their support may be crucial. If they are seen to go through the survey procedures first the people will feel reassured.

In one survey a local politician was not adequately informed and took great trouble to go around and tell people that the survey was a plot to sterilize all the children! In any particular community there are often several subgroups, such as religious or language groups, each with their own set of leaders; offence may be taken if a survey team approaches only some groups or becomes friendly with and appears to side with one faction.

Other medical staff in the area

Sometimes existing medical staff in an area feel threatened by a survey team that comes in from outside. They may fear that they will have an increased workload, or that the survey will reveal unsatisfactory conditions prevailing in their area. Discussion with them before the survey is important because it is often they who interpret the purpose of the survey to the local leaders and population. Where possible local medical staff should join the study. This allows knowledge to be shared between them and the investigators.

Selection of personnel

The survey personnel may themselves arouse adverse reactions in certain cultures and societies. They are often foreign to the area and unable to speak the language, and they may be unaware of the sensitivities of the people. Small things such as a woman doctor wearing trousers or having painted fingernails may be offensive. In many Muslim areas women do not like to be examined by a male doctor and it is then essential to have a woman as a member of the team. Whenever women are to be examined female staff should of course be present.

It is often an advantage if some of the staff are known in the area and have been locally recruited. Language problems must be considered and if the investigators do not speak the language of the population, or if there are several subgroups with different languages, then suitably trained interpreters must be used and must be acceptable to the population. The investigator himself should always know at least the greetings, and it is advisable to carry a list of sentences that will be used frequently.

Laboratory tests

Where laboratory tests are to be undertaken one must consider the reaction of the population. For instance some people object to putting a specimen of faeces in a container, since they believe that an ill-wisher can use something from his victim for bewitchment. Taking blood samples at night to detect filariasis is especially likely to arouse these sort of fears. In one survey people's anxiety was relieved when the examination of the stool specimen was done on the spot and the remains openly discarded into a pit. It is wise to show all containers to be used to the community before the survey. This will ensure nobody is offended.

Many people have fears when they see blood carefully packed and put into thermos flasks to be taken away, especially if they get further reports that it will then be put on an aircraft to be sent to Europe. A common belief is that blood samples are sold. Related to this is the complaint that people are not told the results of tests. Results should be available to people and the outcome of the project should be discussed with the community at large.

Nowadays it is often easier to preserve and transport specimens to a big laboratory rather than attempt to process them under adverse conditions in the field. Therefore containers may become an important item to consider. They must be cheap, durable, and have labels that do not come off or become illegible. Diamond pencils, felt pens, ballpoint pens, lead pencils, wax pencils, stick-on labels, leucoplast labels all have special advantages or disadvantages for particular types of containers or specimens. It is important to label all specimens twice in case one label becomes obscured or falls off.

'Line of flow'

If a survey includes a number of procedures, each done by a different worker, it is advisable to devise a 'line of flow', whereby patients or individuals pass from one 'station' to another and have a different procedure done at each. For example, at Station 1 an interviewer may record basic identifying data and issue a numbered record card: in addition, since the records of children within one family readily become interchanged it may be helpful if the serial number is written on each child's arm with a felt pen, providing this gives no offence. The individual with his form then proceeds to Station 2 where another worker does measurements and records them. Station 3 may be manned by the doctor doing a physical examination: he may suggest some immediate treatment which is done at Station 4, where the record card is retrieved and filed. The individual 'processed' in this way has perhaps had 10 minutes at each station and the whole sequence has taken 40 minutes. If timing can be precisely anticipated appointments may be given, which is an advantage when the population surveyed is employed or in school.

If children are being examined it is wise to have traumatic procedures last. Blood-taking, for example, should come after examination of the skin. A few sweets help to diminish the wailing, and such consideration is appreciated by the mothers, who should accompany their children whenever possible.

Field equipment, housing and transport

Equipment for field surveys has to be carefully listed, as once out in a remote rural area it may be impossible to get an omitted item. It is annoying to find that the diamond pencil for marking the number on glass slides has been forgotten! Each procedure must have a check list of required items, e.g. instruments, diagnostic equipment, containers, forms, reagents, labels. Conditions of storage of specimens may have to be precise and refrigeration at different temperatures may be needed. Gas refrigerators and deep freeze units are available and will operate within Land Rovers or other vehicles. Liquid nitrogen refrigerators may be needed for preserving cells.

It is wise to read detailed accounts of other field studies to discover what particular items of equipment were found most serviceable under field conditions. For example, transistorized audiometers, field centrifuges, small field microscopes, portable generators and field incubators are all available, and some are better suited for particular surveys than others. Spares for all equipment must be carried, and may vary from an extra Heaf gun to a spare bulb for an ophthalmoscope. For some equipment it is wise to anticipate trouble and learn how to do repairs.

Survey 'furniture' may include benches, portable folding tables, screens and examination couches. Much can be improvised: for example, a thin layer of foam rubber on a table with a newspaper sheet will form an adequate couch. 'Safari' equipment for campers and tourists is often ideal for scientific field surveys.

Tents may be necessary if housing is not available but in many countries there are adequate rest houses. It may be convenient to carry out the actual survey procedures in a school or community centre.

For the survey team food supplies, water, personal protection against insect vectors, and appropriate immunization or chemoprophylaxis must be organized.

Transport is always a major item in the budget of a field survey. Sturdy vehicles such as Land Rovers have great appeal and their four-wheel drive may be essential in certain types of terrain or in the wet season. However, they are costly to run and a smaller vehicle such as a saloon car may in fact be sufficient — and much less expensive. The logistics of a survey have to be carefully worked out in advance to avoid unnecessary trips. A check on mileage has also to be maintained as vehicles tend to be used unnecessarily.

EXECUTION

Supervision of staff

Minimization of observer error in epidemiological surveys requires not only careful preliminary training of staff in the use of a particular technique, but also continued supervision throughout the course of the survey, to ensure that the procedures are not varying from the initial standard.

Fieldwork is interesting and exciting but tiring, especially if it is done in areas where the normal routine of the worker is not possible. Three weeks without a shave or a bath, living on an unvarying diet of cassava and beans, is often as much as the staff can take without becoming inexact in their recording. During prolonged field surveys it is useful to return to the nearest town or hotel every 3–4 weeks to review the work that has been done, to put schedules in order, to list data that are missing and still have to be collected, to send specimens to the laboratory and to reorganize supplies.

Continuing discussion with the population

Sometimes a survey begins well, with people presenting themselves in expected numbers, but after a few days attendance falls or ceases altogether. The cause may be a sudden rumour about the purpose of the survey. A sample survey of a community in East Africa was rumoured to be selecting immigrants for repatriation. Another cause may be an unfortunate incident, perhaps a haematoma following a venepuncture, or a coincidental death in the village thought to have been caused by the survey. However, good communication between the population and survey team can go far to forestall and eliminate this kind of difficulty, and may be accomplished by informal discussion with the local people at the end of the day's work. If the survey staff are prepared to stay on after hours to see the chief's sick child, or to share a meal with a villager, this type of rapport will go a long way to maintaining good relationships. The staff should also be prepared to take a few minutes off during the day to discuss misunderstandings which arise; it is important that all staff give the same explanations of their activities and procedures.

In any survey there are always a number of people who fail to attend for interview or examination when requested to do so. There are many reasons for not co-operating, such as illness, unwillingness to participate, or lack of information. Those who do not co-operate may be an important group whose exclusion from the survey will bias the results. They may, for example, include a disproportionate number of people who are severely affected by the disease being studied, and who, for this reason, are unable to travel to the survey centre. It is therefore necessary to have a system for finding non-attenders and encouraging them or assisting them to attend.

In longitudinal descriptive studies or cohort studies, in which repeated observations are made on the same group of people during many months or years, the problems of ensuring continued co-operation are accentuated and always require careful thought by the investigator. Here in particular on-going results and difficulties need to be discussed with the community. The use of visual methods such as flannel graphs, slides and films may help to clarify the purpose of the study.

It may be tempting to take photographs at all stages of a survey to ensure a complete record of the procedures. However, people often resent being photographed by an unknown investigator. When the investigators are well known, and if permission is asked, then photography may even be enjoyed, especially if a Polaroid camera is used and some photographs are given away.

8. Analysis and presentation of findings

ANALYSIS

In general the purpose of an analysis is to extract from a mass of information a few numerical statements which fairly summarize the data. Numerical data may be considered under two headings: in *binary data* only the presence or absence of a characteristic is recorded, with no statement of magnitude, for example the presence or absence of leprosy or of a palpable spleen; whereas *quantitative data* are derived from measurements on a scale and therefore comprise numbers on the particular scale being used, for example haemoglobin concentrations in g/100 ml.

Binary data

A simple example of binary data derived in an epidemiological study is a count of the number of persons in a population sample who have or do not have a palpable spleen.

When counts are made from a large number of survey records a tallying method is useful. One simple method is that in which each count of 1 is represented by a vertical line, and 4 counts are joined by a horizontal line to make a unit of 5. Thus |||| |||| || represents 12.

Suppose a count shows that out of 90 boys examined in a survey 24 were recorded as having a palpable spleen while in 66 the spleen was impalpable. Usually an observation of this kind would be made with the purpose of comparing it with a similar observation on another group of children. Suppose then that among 120 girls coming from the same area as the 90 males it is found that 44 have palpable spleens whilst 76 do not. This type of data will usually be set out in what is known as a 2 × 2 table, shown in Table 8.1.

The 2 × 2 table is widely used in epidemiology as a concise

Table 8.1 Numbers of children with and without palpable spleens

Sex	With palpable spleen	Without palpable spleen	Totals
Boys	24	66	90
Girls	44	76	120
Totals	68	142	210

method of presenting results. It is easy to comprehend and to analyse statistically. The totals of the columns and rows should always be included, to make nine 'cells' of figures in the table.

In analysing the data in this table, in order to compare the counts of palpable spleens among boys and girls, it is usual to express the number of palpable spleens in each group as a percentage of the total. Thus 27% (24/90) of boys have palpable spleens compared with 37% (44/120) of girls, and it is concluded that palpable spleens are more frequent among females than males in the group of children examined. In most circumstances such a conclusion is of little interest unless it can be generalized to relate to a larger group of children than the 210 actually examined. Usually the two groups of boys and girls would have been drawn as samples from a defined study population (Ch. 3). Provided that the samples were drawn by a random procedure observations made on them may be formally related to the study population.

The rates of 27 and 37% observed in boys and girls are sample estimates of the rates in the study population and are associated with sampling errors. Because only this inexact estimate of the population rates is available one cannot conclude with certainty that female rates are greater than male rates in the population. It is possible that in the population the rates are the same or even that male rates are higher than female, but that the operation of chance factors in sample selection has given the observed lower rate in males.

Suppose that instead of spleen rates of 27% in boys and 37% in girls one has observed rates of 10% in boys and 70% in girls (in sample of 90 boys and 120 girls as before). The investigator will feel more confident that male rates are lower than female rates in the population from which the samples were drawn. This increased confidence results from an awareness that the larger the difference in spleen rates observed in the two samples of the population, the less likely it is that those two samples were drawn from a population in which male and female rates are identical.

Significance tests

By relating the magnitude of a difference observed, such as that between male and female spleen rates, to the size of the samples taken, significance tests such as the χ^2 test quantify the frequency with which the observed difference, or a larger one, would occur in a series of samples of the particular size, drawn from a population in which male and female spleen rates were in fact the same. The results of significance tests are expressed in relation to a scale of probability (P). If, for example, a result of $P = 0.01$ is obtained this would indicate that the difference observed between male and female spleen rates, or a larger difference, would occur on average in only 1 out of every 100 samples of that size drawn from a population in which the rates were the same. Since an event which is predicted to occur only once in every 100 occasions is an unusual event, the investigator may choose to say that the results are unlikely to be a consequence of such an unusual event, and are more likely to result from sampling of a population in which female rates exceed male rates. On the other hand if significance tests give a P value of 0.1 this indicates that the observed difference, or a larger one, in male and female spleen rates would occur on 1 in 10 occasions when samples of that size are drawn from a population in which male and female rates are the same. In these circumstances the investigator may decide that it is not unlikely that the difference observed in the male and female samples is only the result of chance factors operating in sample selection, and he may be unwilling to conclude that male and female rates in the population are different.

By convention if P is less than 0.05 the results are said to be *statistically significant*, and would tend to support a decision by the investigator that the results reflect a real difference between male and female spleen rates in the population rather than an apparent difference due to chance factors in sampling.

It is suggested that a reader wishing to use significance tests refers to a book on statistical methods such as those mentioned in Suggested Further Reading. For the purposes of this chapter it is sufficient to make one important point. An investigator must not adopt a slavish attitude to significance tests, accepting all differences between samples with P of less than 0.05 as indicating differences in the population being sampled, and rejecting those with

P values of more than 0.05. A decision about the interpretation of results must be made primarily in the light of existing biological knowledge. It is the responsibility of the investigator to consider the relevant biological facts in relation to the statistical evidence from his own results and make a decision about the interpretation of the results. If the investigator, with his intimate knowledge of the problem and the conditions under which the data were collected, cannot interpret his results it is perhaps unlikely that anyone else can do so for him. Generally it is improper merely to express a finding in terms of a value for P without expressing any opinion as to whether this reflects a characteristic of the population being studied or merely the vagaries of the sampling procedure. Further confirmation of the findings of a survey must often come from repeated surveys on other populations.

The interpretation of Table 8.1 is simple in that the investigator must choose between two alternatives, for the observed difference in male and female spleen rates is due either to sampling variation or to differences between the spleen rates in the population consequent upon exposure or reaction either to malaria or possibly to some other disorder. For a 2 × 2 table which showed that oesophageal cancer was more common among maize-eating peoples than non-maize-eating peoples the interpretation would be more complex. First the investigator must enquire whether the association is the result of bias, for example better ascertainment of oesophageal cancer in the maize-eating communities. Secondly, having discounted bias — a process which may demand exhaustive inquiry and analysis — he must choose between the alternatives of (1) sampling variation; (2) a maize diet is a determinant of oesophageal cancer; (3) a maize diet and oesophageal cancer are associated because the occurrence of both depends upon some third and unknown influence, such as climate. Put in general terms, when data suggest that two variables or attributes A and B are associated, the possible explanations are (1) bias; (2) sampling variation; (3) A is a determinant of B; (4) B is a determinant of A; (5) A and B are determined by common variables; (6) some combination of the foregoing explanations. The choice between possibilities (3) and (4) does not usually present much difficulty.

Analysis of pairs

In an analytic study in which the controls have been selected by matched-pairing with individuals in the study group, analysis of the results depends upon comparison of the individuals within each pair rather than comparison of the overall rates in the study and control groups. For a discussion of this type of analysis the reader is referred to the book by Kirkwood (see Suggested Further Reading, p. 170).

Quantitative data

Frequency distributions

Table 8.2 shows the number of children in each of 100 families. It may be seen that there are more families with three children than with any other number. There are also many families with one, two, four and five children, but fewer with no children or six or more. This tabulation is an example of a frequency distribution. Epidemiological data are often tabulated in the form of such distributions, which show the frequency with which different values or ranges of values of a variable occur in a series of observations.

Table 8.2 Frequency distribution of 100 families according to number of children

Number of children in family	Frequency (no. of families)
0	9
1	13
2	15
3	17
4	14
5	10
6	6
7	5
8	4
9	2
10	2
11	0
12	2
13	1
Total	100

If the value of a variable changes by whole numbers, for example counts of children in a family, the variable is known as *discrete*, to distinguish it from a *continuous* variable in which fractional values occur, for example blood urea levels. If a discrete variable has a wide range of values, it will be necessary to *group* the values before constructing a frequency distribution. Table 8.3 shows the distribution of white blood cell counts among 89 adult men attending a health centre. The counts have been grouped in intervals of 2000

Table 8.3   Frequency distribution of white blood cell counts per mm^3

White blood cell	Frequency
2000−	7
4000−	24
6000−	22
8000−	16
10 000−	12
12 000−	5
14 000−	1
16 000+	2
Total	89

and the data thereby compressed to a frequency distribution comprising eight groups. The investigator is free to choose any interval of grouping depending on the number of observations, but an interval which gives somewhere between five and 15 groupings is often the most suitable. Less than five groupings compresses the pattern of the distribution excessively, and with more than 15 the number of observations in each group may become so small that the pattern of the distribution is obscured. The groups must always be defined in such a way that each value of the variable can only be assigned to one group. A grouping of age, recorded to the nearest year, into 0–5, 5–10, 10–15, 15 and over is incorrect since people aged 5, 10 and 15 can be assigned to two groups. A correct grouping is 0–4, 5–9, 10–14, 15 and over.

A continuous variable must usually be grouped before a frequency distribution can be constructed, because each value in, for example, a series of haemoglobin concentrations measured to one decimal place may be unique in that series. Grouping of the haemoglobin values at a suitable interval such as 2 g/100 ml (i.e. 4.0–5.9, 6.0–7.9, 8.0–9.9 . . .) enables a frequency distribution to be tabulated.

Data tabulated as a frequency distribution may be displayed graphically as a *frequency polygon*. Some examples of these have already been given. Figure 8.1 shows a frequency polygon of the data given in Table 8.3. The frequency in each group is represented by a point at a corresponding height above the horizontal axis. The points are joined by straight lines. Figure 8.1 illustrates the form of most frequency polygons seen in epidemiological work, having a single peak, known as the *mode*, from which the line falls away on either side. It may be noted that the shape of the polygon is not symmetrical, and this asymmetry is commonly seen in biological

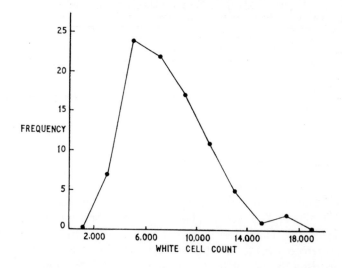

Fig. 8.1 Frequency distribution of white blood cell counts in 89 adult men.

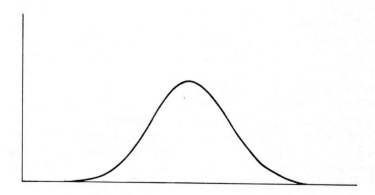

Fig. 8.2 The normal distribution.

distributions. The form of the polygon in Figure 8.1 may be compared to that in Figure 8.2 which shows a symmetrical curve known as a *normal curve*. Many distributions in biology approximate to a normal curve, although few have its exact form. The normal distribution is of central importance in statistical theory and will be referred to later in this chapter.

Table 8.4   Weights (kg) of 35 8-year-old boys

23	21	26	27	22	20	24
24	23	23	18	24	22	22
22	20	22	29	26	25	27
23	21	22	20	24	24	21
22	21	16	19	18	25	23

Summarizing indices

At the end of a survey in which quantitative data are recorded the investigator is confronted with a series of measurements, such as the weights of 35 8-year-old boys attending a health centre, shown in Table 8.4. These measurements must be compared with similar measurements made in other surveys, and in order to make this comparison the salient features of the data must be summarized in a few indices.

The *arithmetic mean*, or average, is the most commonly used index and is obtained by adding all the measurements and dividing the sum by the number of measurements. The mean must be distinguished from two other indices which are sometimes used, the *median* and the *mode*. The median is the middle of a series of values arranged in order of magnitude. In the series of 7 values: 6, 11, 12, 15, 19, 24, 35 the median is the fourth value 15, since half of the values exceed it and half are below it. If there are an even number of values in a series the median is conventionally taken as the average of the middle two values. Although not as frequently used as the mean the median has particular applications. In describing the survival times of cancer patients after therapy the median gives a better reflection of prognosis than the mean, since the latter is unduly influenced by a few patients with long survival.

The mode of a frequency distribution is the value which occurs with the highest frequency. In Table 8.3 the modal group is 4000.

The mean of the weights listed in Table 8.4 is 22.5 kg. But this is an inadequate description of the data since many of the weights differ markedly from the mean. The *range* of the values is from 16 to 29. But this again is an inadequate description since it defines only the two extreme values in the series.

The variation within a series of observations is best summarized by calculation of the *standard deviation* which is a measure of the scatter of the observations around their mean. The stages in the calculation of the standard deviation are as follows:

1. The difference between the value of each observation and the mean is calculated. Thus in Table 8.4 the difference for the first observation, 23, is (23–22.5) = 0.5

2. Each of the differences is squared.

3. The squares are added and the total is divided by the number of observations minus 1. For Table 8.4 the resultant is 7.55.

4. The square root of the resultant gives the standard deviation, which is 2.75.

The standard deviation is dependent upon the average deviation of each observation from the mean of all the observations. In practice it is calculated by methods which are quicker than the one described and avoid the tedious subtraction of the mean from each of a large series of observations. Sophisticated desk calculators are now widely available and enable the calculation to be done simply and speedily.

A large standard deviation shows that there is a wide scatter of observations around the mean value, while a small standard deviation shows that the observations are concentrated around the mean with little variation between one observation and another. It may be noted that of the 35 body weights only the two extreme values (16 and 29) fall outside the range of the mean plus or minus twice the standard deviation (22.5 ± 2 × 2.75 = 17–28).

Use of mean and standard deviation

The mean and standard deviation are the two usual indices used to summarize a series of measurements. However, they cannot be used automatically for all measurements since they are unsuitable when a frequency distribution differs markedly from the normal curve (Fig. 8.2). The distribution of size of reactions to Mantoux testing with 5 TU, shown in Figure 8.3, has two peaks at 2–4 mm and 16–18 mm. This distribution is bimodal (having two modes or peaks) and the mean and standard deviation would be inappropriate summarizing indices.

Bimodal distributions

Figure 8.4 shows the interesting age distribution of female deaths from kuru (the distribution is drawn in the form of a histogram, described in a later section of this chapter). Whereas age distributions of diseases usually have a single peak or modal value this distribution is clearly bimodal; deaths from kuru are most frequent

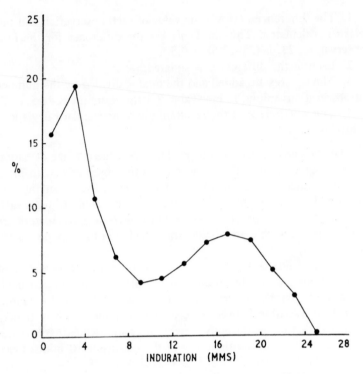

Fig. 8.3 Percentage distribution of size in induration after 5 TU Mantoux test (5915 people in Uganda).

among 5–9-year-old and 20–39-year-old females. This bimodality seems to result from differing exposure to the causative virus in different age-groups, with women and young children having the highest exposure. The interpretation of bimodal distributions has received much attention in epidemiology. The bimodal age distribution of Hodgkin's disease in North America, for example, has led to the hypothesis that the disease comprises two distinct disorders, with differing aetiology, one affecting young people and the other older people. However, there are two points relating to bimodal distributions which make their interpretation difficult. First, inaccuracies of measurement or recording, and small numbers of observations, are a frequent source of bimodality in distributions which truly have one mode. Secondly, two frequency distributions, with different modes, often do not make a bimodal distribution when combined together; the absence of bimodality does not signify that the data have come from a homogeneous source.

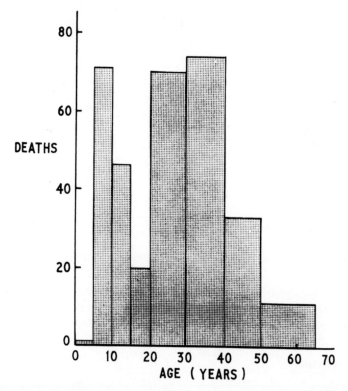

Fig. 8.4   Age distribution of deaths from kuru among females, 1957–1959.
From: Alpers M, Gajdusek D C 1965 American Journal of Tropical Medicine
and Hygiene 14: 852.

Significance tests

In the section describing analysis of binary data it was shown that
measurements of rates, such as spleen rates, in a sample gave an
imprecise estimate of spleen rates in the population, because a single random sample is unlikely to be exactly representative of the
population from which it is drawn. For the same reason the values
of a series of quantitative measurements made on a sample and
summarized as the mean and standard deviation are not exact estimates of the values in the population. Using the same arguments
as were applied to binary data, tests of significance may be used
to determine whether observed differences between series of measurements made on two or more samples are statistically significant.
The tests of significance used include calculation of the *standard*

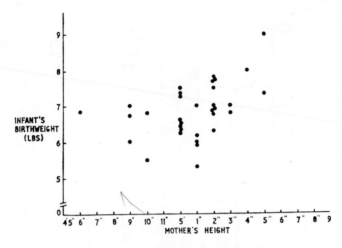

Fig. 8.5 Birthweights of 33 female infants and mothers' heights.

error of the difference of the means, and comparison of two means by the *t-test.* Again the reader is referred to one of the books on statistical methods mentioned in Suggested Further Reading.

Correlation

Figure 8.5 shows measurements of the birthweights of 33 female infants plotted against the heights of their mothers. Each dot corresponds to the height of a mother, plotted along the horizontal axis, and the birthweight of her child, plotted along the vertical axis. The 33 dots correspond to the 33 mother-and-baby pairs. It may be seen that taller mothers tend to have heavier babies and therefore the two variables, mother's height and infant's birthweight, are said to be *correlated.* When two variables are correlated an increase or decrease in one is associated with an increase or decrease in the other. Figure 8.6 shows hypothetical data in which mother's height and infant's birthweight are not correlated, being independent of one another.

Figure 8.5 is an example of a *scatter diagram,* which may be plotted when paired measurements are made of two variables. From inspection of a scatter diagram an assessment can be made as to whether two variables are correlated and, if so, the degree of correlation between them. Figure 8.7 shows hypothetical data in which there is complete correlation between the birthweight and maternal height, so that knowledge of the mother's height enables precise

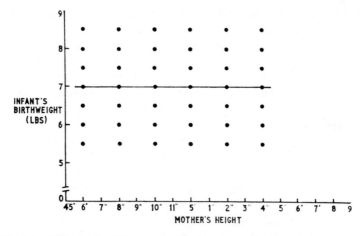

Fig. 8.6 Birthweights of infants and mothers' heights: hypothetical data showing absence of correlation.

prediction of the child's birthweight. In Figure 8.5 the correlation is only partial, for not all the heaviest babies are born to the tallest mothers and vice versa. The degree of correlation between two variables can be quantitated by calculation of the *correlation coefficient*. This coefficient (whose value ranges between +1 and −1) may only be used if inspection of the scatter diagram shows that the relationship between the two variables is adequately described by a straight line. Inspection of Figure 8.5 shows that the relationship of

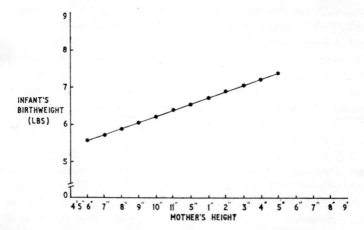

Fig. 8.7 Birthweights of infants and mothers' heights: hypothetical data showing complete correlation.

birthweight and maternal height is approximately linear and there-fore the correlation coefficient may be used.

It has already been pointed out that an *association* between two variables (such as that between the incidence of pellagra and the maize content of the diet) does not necessarily imply that the one variable is a cause of the other. Similarly correlation does not imply a causal relationship. Recent increases in the annual incidence of gonorrhoea in some countries are correlated with increases in the number of traffic accidents. Clearly neither increase causes the other, although both may be reflections of some other change such as increasing urbanization. When a scatter diagram shows two vari-ables to be correlated the investigator seeks to determine whether the correlation results from influences which determine correspond-ing changes in both variables, or from the influence of one variable on the other. When considering maternal height and infant's birthweight it is evident that maternal height could directly influ-ence the size of the baby, but the baby's weight could not influence the mother's height. The birthweight is therefore said to be *depen-dent* on maternal height. When one variable is dependent on an-other the association may be described by the *regression coefficient* which, like the correlation coefficient, assumes a linear relationship between the two variables.

Standardization

Table 8.5 shows the numbers of cases of a disease which occurred within two populations, called A and B, during a specified period of time. Both populations comprise 10 000 individuals and in popu-lation A there were 125 cases while in B there were 182. The in-cidence of the disease is 12.5 per 1000 in A and 18.2 per 1000 in

Table 8.5 Numbers of cases occurring in populations A and B

Population		Age-group (years)			Totals
		0–4	5–14	15+	
A	No. cases	63	50	12	125
	No. population	1500	2500	6000	10 000
	Incidence per 1000	42	20	2	12.5
B	No. cases	90	84	8	182
	No. population	2500	3500	4000	10 000
	Incidence per 1000	36	24	2	18.2

B, and B therefore has an incidence approximately one and a half times greater than A. However, further inspection of the table reveals two facts. First the incidence of the disease varies markedly between the three age-groups, being highest in very young children of 0–4 years and lowest among adults. Secondly the age distributions of the two populations are dissimilar, since B has a greater proportion of young people. Therefore although B has more cases and a higher incidence than A, this may be the result of the different age structures of the two populations, rather than a difference in the levels of exposure or susceptibility to the disease determinants. To solve this problem a procedure known as *direct standardization* may be used, whereby the incidence in each population is adjusted to allow for the difference in age structure. There are three steps in this procedure.

1. For both populations the incidence is calculated within each age-group. This is shown in Table 8.5 where the age-specific incidence for 0–4-year-olds in A, for example, is $63/1500 = 42$ per 1000.

2. A population with a 'standard' age distribution is selected to replace A and B. Although any standard population may be selected its age distribution should approximate that of A and B, and it is convenient to use one or other of them or their sum. In Table 8.6 the two populations have been added to give a standard population (A + B) of 20 000.

3. The age-specific incidences in A and B are multiplied by the standard population numbers, giving standardized numbers of cases. Among 0–4-year-olds in A, for example, the standardized number of cases is $(42 \times 4000)/1000 = 168$. It may be seen that the total of standardized numbers of cases in both A and B is 308, giving an *age-standardized incidence* of $308/20\ 000 = 15.4$ per 1000

Table 8.6 Numbers of cases resulting from application of incidences in A and B to standard population

	Age-group (years)			Totals
	0–4	5–14	15+	
No. standard population (A + B)	4000	6000	10 000	20 000
No. cases in A	168	120	20	308
No. cases in B	144	144	20	308

for each population. Therefore the difference between the unstandardized or *crude incidence* rates of 12.5 and 18.2 per 1000 in A and B is solely attributable to their different age-structures.

The foregoing example shows why, as stated in Chapter 2, comparison of morbidity and mortality in different populations requires calculation of standardized rates. It is usual to standardize for sex as well as age, the procedure being identical to that described with the addition that numbers of cases in the standard population are calculated for males and females separately and then combined to give an *age/sex-standardized rate*.

When morbidity and mortality rates are standardized the investigator is free to choose any population as the standard. In the fore going example the sum of the two populations A and B was used, but another standard such as the population of the particular region or country would be acceptable. However, the choice of standard will influence the comparison. For example, it has been shown that when three different standards commonly used in international comparisons of cancer morbidity are applied to the comparison of gastric cancer incidence in England and Nigeria, they give excess incidences in England of respectively, 60, 90 and 109%. The investigator is therefore wise to choose a standard which is also used by others working in the same field.

In the technique of direct standardization which has been described the 'standard' used is the age/sex structure of a chosen population. The alternative technique, that of *indirect standardization*, depends upon the use of standard age/sex-specific rates. Applying this technique to the data in Table 8.5 it is convenient to use as a standard the combined incidence rates for populations A and B. These rates are shown in Table 8.7, where the combined incidences are 38.2, 22.3, and 2.0 for the three age-groups. These

Table 8.7 Numbers of cases resulting from application of standard incidence to populations A and B

	Age-group (years)			Totals
	0–4	5–14	15+	
Standard incidence per 1000 (incidence in A + B)	38.2	22.3	2.0	–
No. cases in A	57	56	12	125
No. cases in B	96	78	8	182

rates are applied separately to populations A and B to give an expected number of cases in each age-group. The totals of the expected numbers of cases are identical to those actually observed, i.e. 125 for A and 182 for B. This again demonstrates that the difference in crude incidence rates in A and B is solely attributable to their different age structures.

Similarly to direct standardization the investigator using indirect standardization is free to choose any standard, but the choice will influence the comparison of the populations to which the standard rates are applied. The Registrar General in England and Wales uses indirect standardization to compare annual mortality rates in different regions. The age/sex-specific death rates for the total population are used as the standard and applied to each region. The resulting expected number of deaths in a given region is compared with the number which actually occurred. The comparison is expressed as the *standardized mortality ratio* (SMR) which is the product of (no. of deaths which occurred × 100)/(no. of expected deaths). If the SMR exceeds 100 the mortality experienced by that region is higher than that for the country as a whole after allowing for the age/sex structure of the region. Likewise an SMR below 100 indicates a lower mortality than for the country as a whole.

Generally indirect standardization is used instead of direct if the numbers of cases in the age/sex-groups of the population being studied are too small to give reliable age/sex-specific rates.

The use of standardization techniques is not confined to comparison of morbidity and mortality in different populations. Tables 8.8 and 8.9 show the distribution of cases of mycobacterial skin ulcers by age, sex, and site of lesion in two case series from different areas of Uganda. In series 1, 48 out of 84 (57%) of the lesions were on the legs rather than any other part of the body. In series 2 only 36 out of 87 (41%) of the lesions were on the legs. It is thought that mycobacterial ulcers occur at the site where the organism is inoculated into the skin by some, at present unknown, environmental agency. If in two different areas of Uganda the distribution of lesions on the body differs this suggests that the nature of transmission of the infection may also differ. However, inspection of Tables 8.8 and 8.9 shows that the proportion of ulcers occurring on the legs differs in different age- and sex-groups. Leg ulcers are more common among males than females and more common among older males than younger males. Series 1, which has the greater proportion of leg ulcers, also has the higher ratio of males to females and a higher ratio of older to younger males. Part at least of the

Table 8.8 Mycobacterial skin ulcers, series 1

Site of lesions	Males				Females				Males and females
	Age-group (years)			All males	Age-group (years)			All females	
	0–9	10–14	15+		0–9	10–14	15+		
Legs	12 (10.6)	12 (7.5)	13 (7.2)	37	4 (6.6)	2 (3.6)	5 (6.8)	11	48 (42)
Other sites	9 (8.0)	6 (3.8)	3 (1.6)	18	7 (11.5)	4 (7.2)	7 (9.4)	18	36 (42)
All sites	21 (18.6)	18 (11.3)	16 (8.8)	55	11 (18.1)	6 (10.8)	12 (16.2)	29	84

Figures in brackets are derived by standardization: see text.

Table 8.9 Mycobacterial skin ulcers, series 2

Site of lesions	Males				Females				Males and females
	Age-group (years)			All males	Age-group (years)			All females	
	0–9	10–14	15+		0–9	10–14	15+		
Legs	8 (9.1)	3 (7.0)	2 (9.1)	13	9 (6.5)	5 (3.5)	9 (7.2)	23	36 (42)
Other sites	9 (10.2)	2 (4.7)	0	11	17 (12.3)	11 (7.7)	12 (9.6)	40	51 (45)
All sites	17 (19.3)	5 (11.7)	2 (9.1)	24	26 (18.8)	16 (11.2)	21 (16.8)	63	87

Figures in brackets are derived by standardization: see text.

excess of leg ulcers in series 1, in comparison with series 2, can therefore be accounted for by the age and sex distribution of the cases. But, having allowed for the differences in age/sex distribution, does there remain any difference in distribution of site of lesion in the two series?

To answer this point one may use a simple standardization procedure similar to the direct technique already described. A standard age/sex distribution is applied to both series. This standard may be derived by addition of the two series so that 0–9-year-old males, for example, comprise $(21 + 17) = 38$ out of a total of $(84 + 87) = 171$, which equals 22.2%. Application of the standard percentage distribution to each series is effected by multiplication of the standard by the total number of cases in the series. Thus the standardized number of 0–9-year-old males in series 1 is $(22.2 \times 84) = 18.6$ and in series 2 is $(22.2 \times 87) = 19.3$. (It is more precise to retain a decimal place at this stage of the calculation.) The standardized numbers of cases are then distributed between the two sites, 'legs' or 'other sites', in the proportion of the unstandardized observations. Among 0–9-year-old males in series 1 there were 12 out of 21 lesions on the legs. Among the 18.6 standardized cases there will be $(12 \times 18.6)/21 = 10.6$ leg lesions. In this way calculation is made of the number of leg and other site lesions within each age/sex-group which would be expected if the standard age/sex distribution applied to each series. The expected numbers, which are shown in brackets in Tables 8.8 and 8.9, are then totalled giving 42 leg lesions out of 84 in series 1 and 42 out of 87 in series 2. Therefore after standardization for age and sex there is little difference between the site of lesions in the two series. (It may be noted that the difference in age/sex distribution of the two case series in the example is somewhat greater than is usually found in two case series of the same disease.)

Simple standardization techniques of this kind are often used in epidemiological analyses. Sometimes more complex techniques, such as *multiple regression analysis*, are used, and the extensive calculations which are involved usually necessitate a computer. In general when a variable or attribute being studied is influenced by a number of other variables or attributes, standardization techniques enable determination of the magnitude of the influence of one variable or attribute after allowing for the influence of the others.

Standardization gives an overall figure for the number of leg ulcers expected in each series allowing for the age/sex distribution.

Table 8.10 Ratio of leg/other site lesions in series 1 and 2

	Males (years)			Females (years)		
	0–9	10–14	15+	0–9	10–14	15+
Series 1	1.3	2.0	4.3	0.6	0.5	0.7
Series 2	0.9	1.5	$(\frac{2}{0})$	0.5	0.4	0.7

But a 'standardized' comparison could also be made by considering the ratio of leg to other site lesions in the two series within each age/sex-group. This comparison (Table 8.10) shows that the ratios in the two series are similar, and suggests the overall excess of leg lesions in series 1 is due to the age/sex distribution. Comparison within each subgroup is more informative and therefore preferable if the numbers in each subgroup are large; but if the numbers are small, as in the example given, an overall standardized figure may give the most suitable basis for comparison.

In analytic studies practical difficulties in the selection of a study or control group, or subsequent loss of individuals from one or other group because of migration, lack of co-operation or some other reason, sometimes results in unavoidable differences in the distribution of some important variable or attribute in the two groups. At other times the importance of a variable or attribute only comes to light during analysis, when it is too late to match the study and control groups. In either of these circumstances standardization corrects for dissimilarities in the study and control groups and enables their comparison; it must be emphasized however that this procedure cannot be used as a substitute for the careful initial selection of controls in accordance with the principles described in Chapter 4.

PRESENTATION OF FINDINGS

Written reports

When the results of investigations are reported it is usual to set them out in five sections:

1. *Introduction*, in which the purpose of the investigation is described.

2. *Methods*, in which the population studied and the techniques used are described.
3. *Results*, in which the findings of the investigation are presented.
4. *Discussion*, in which the interpretation of the findings is discussed.
5. *Summary*, in which the essence of the investigation is summarized.

In the Results section the findings are usually presented as tabulations or diagrams whose main features are also described in the text. Choice of the most appropriate tables and diagrams is critical, both because they enable the investigator to describe the findings concisely and because they may suggest to him some aspects of the data which he has not yet analysed. Each table or diagram should be designed to demonstrate only one or two points, for it is usually better to have a number of simple tables or diagrams than a single complex one. They should be self-explanatory and comprehensible without reference to the accompanying text. The heading should indicate the precise source of the data including the population, the place and the date. Although a simple and concise presentation of findings is essential it may be helpful to other investigators in the same field if the full results of a survey are available for scrutiny. To meet this requirement it is sometimes possible to publish additional numerical data as an appendix to the main report.

Tabulation

A tabulation is the simplest method of setting out numerical data. It should summarize the important features of the data and should have as few figures as is compatible with this objective. If the table comprises figures such as percentages, which are derived by calculation from the original observations, they should be accompanied by sufficient data to enable recalculation of the original numbers. Percentages, rates and other derived figures should not be expressed with more precision, for example to more decimal places, than is compatible with the precision of the original observations.

Since most epidemiological data can be summarized in tabulations it is helpful if, at the beginning of an investigation, the investigator defines the tabulations he wishes to make. This ensures that the objectives of the investigation are precisely defined at the outset.

Line diagrams

The frequency polygons shown in Figures 3.1, 5.4–5.6 and 8.1–8.3 are examples of line diagrams, the simplest and most frequently used method of displaying epidemiological data.

In line diagrams it is usual for the scale of the vertical axis to begin at zero. If the range of values on this axis is so large that it cannot be fitted on to a scale which begins at zero the axis is interrupted by a space so that the reader's attention is drawn to this fact (as in Fig. 8.5). Adjacent points on a diagram must be joined by straight and not curved lines. Extension of the line beyond the two extreme points at either end is known as extrapolation and is incorrect.

For the study of *rates of change* in a variable, for example the rate of decline in smallpox mortality following initiation of a vaccination campaign, line diagrams may be plotted on *logarithmic scales*. These logarithmic plots are made on specially prepared paper on which either the vertical axis alone has a logarithmic scale (giving a semilogarithmic plot) or both the vertical and horizontal axes have logarithmic scales. Plotting the values of a variable on a logarithmic scale is equivalent to taking the logarithm of each value and plotting it on a conventional scale. When a variable is plotted on a logarithmic scale a constant rate of change is indicated by a straight line whose slope is proportional to the rate.

Figure 8.8 shows the rise in the numbers of cases of AIDS in Oceania since 1982, plotted on a conventional scale. The graph shows that the number of cases increased steeply. In Figure 8.9 the same data are plotted on a semi-logarithmic scale. The slope of the line become progressively flatter, showing that the rate of increase in incidence is declining.

Histograms

Frequency distributions can be represented by frequency polygons, as already described, or by histograms, of which an example is shown in Figure 8.4. The frequency of deaths from kuru in each age-group is represented by the *area* of the corresponding rectangle. If the ages had been grouped in equal intervals the width of each rectangle would be the same, and the numbers of deaths in each age-group would be proportional to the *heights* of the rectangle. However, unequal groupings have been used and the width of the rectangle for the 10 year age-group, 20–29 years, has to be twice

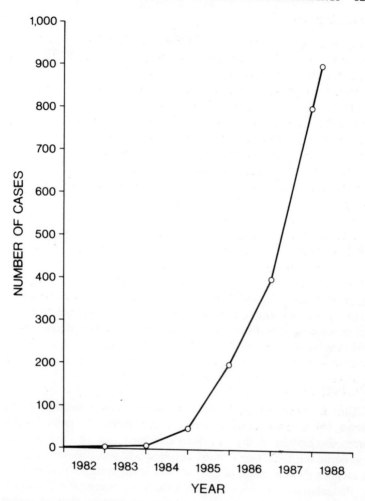

Fig. 8.8 Annual numbers of cases of AIDS in Oceania (plotted on a conventional scale).

that of the 5 year group, 5–9 years. Therefore although the heights of the rectangles for these two groups are the same the area for the 10 year age-group, 20–29 years, has to be twice that of the 5 year group, 5–9 years indicating that there were twice as many deaths in the former as in the latter.

Bar diagrams

In a bar diagram magnitudes are represented by proportional

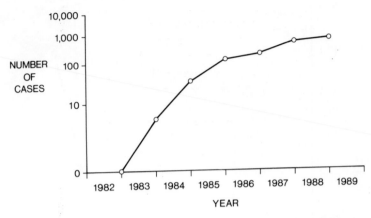

Fig. 8.9 Annual numbers of cases of AIDS in Oceania (plotted on a semi-logarithmic scale).

lengths of bars. Figure 8.10 shows the life expectancy at birth in selected places. Unlike the histogram the width of each bar is of no consequence, and the life expectancies are represented solely by the lengths of the bars.

Pie diagrams

Figure 8.11 is a so-called 'pie' diagram representing the relative frequency of four kinds of serological response to polio vaccine given to children in West Africa. The 'pies' are the circles which represent the total numbers of children and are divided into sections such that the angle of each section at the centre is proportional to the relative frequency of each kind of response. Pie charts are easy to comprehend and are useful when numerical data are being presented to audiences unaccustomed to interpreting scientific results.

Maps

Mapping out the distribution of a disease is a fascinating and often unexpectedly rewarding task. The map in the doctor's office soon becomes covered in an array of different coloured pins and labels on which he is able to reflect at leisure. But maps prepared for publication must usually be simplified, as is shown in Figure 8.12. To make this map of the prevalence of Bancroftian filariasis in

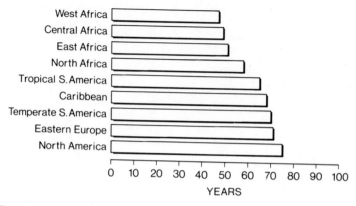

Fig. 8.10 Life expectancy at birth in selected places in 1988.

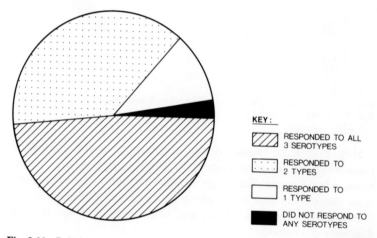

Fig. 8.11 Relative frequency of serological response to three type of polio vaccine.

Tanzania the percentage of adult males infected was recorded in 150 villages throughout the country. The percentages were put into four groupings: (1) less than 6; (2) 6–29; (3) 30–45; (4) more than 45. Each grouping is represented on the map by a different kind of shading. Comparison of such a map with maps showing climatic, geological, biological and other distributions may reveal influences which determine disease distribution. Bancroftian filariasis in Tanzania is found to be rare above 1000 metres and in dry areas; prevalence is positively correlated with temperature and humidity.

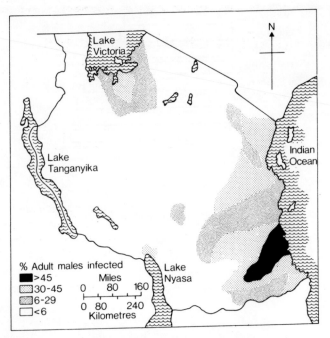

Fig. 8.12 Prevalence of Bancroftian filariasis in Tanzania. From Berry L 1971 Tanzania in maps. London University Press, London.

If the data to be presented are complex, such as the incidence of three forms of cancer in each of 10 districts, then it is preferable to use a bar diagram. But an investigator should not be discouraged from simplifying data and making an additional presentation as a map, for maps stimulate ideas and hypotheses in a way that bar diagrams do not.

9. Investigation of epidemics

INFECTIOUS DISEASE EPIDEMICS

Epidemics of infectious disease, such as cholera, meningococcal meningitis, typhoid, typhus and plague, are an important threat in many tropical countries, and in the past profoundly influenced European history. Modern epidemiology arose out of the study of such classical epidemics, with outbreaks of disease affecting many people and caused by infections, or in some instances dietary deficiency or poisoning.

A general distinction is made between point-source and contagious disease epidemics. In a *point-source epidemic* many susceptible individuals are exposed, more or less simultaneously, to a source of pathogenic organisms or toxins, as when guests at a feast eat meat contaminated with staphylococci. The result of such exposure is an explosive increase in the number of cases of disease over a short period. The time-pattern of a point-source epidemic is illustrated in Figure 5.4. It may be compared with that of a *contagious disease epidemic*, illustrated in Figure 5.5, when organisms are propagated in the community by passage from person to person, so that the initial rise in the number of cases is less abrupt than in point-source epidemics.

The distinction between point-source and contagious disease epidemics is not always clear-cut. A prostitute may be the point-source in a gonorrhoea outbreak, but since she will infect her clients over a period of time there may be no explosive rise in the number of cases.

A feature of developing countries is the multiplicity of endemic communicable diseases, such as typhoid, hepatitis, sleeping sickness, plague, and kala-azar. The term *endemic* implies the habitual presence of a disease or agent of disease within a given area. Levels of endemicity may be defined; for malaria the terms hypoendemic, mesoendemic, hyperendemic, and holoendemic define increasing levels of prevalence as estimated by surveys of spleen and parasite rates in particular age-groups.

Many endemic diseases rapidly become epidemic if environmental or host influences change in a way which favours transmission. Sometimes ecological changes favour the breeding of an insect vector, or there may be an accumulation of non-immune persons in a population either by births or by immigration from a non-endemic area. At other times an epidemic may be heralded by an increase in the organism in carriers or animals. In plague, for instance, an *epizootic* (an epidemic in animals) occurs in rats before an epidemic begins in a human population.

MODERN EPIDEMICS

In current usage the term *epidemic* is applied to any pronounced rise in incidence or prevalence rates and is not restricted to sudden outbreaks. The time period is no longer confined to weeks or months. Slow epidemics of leprosy, spread over several generations, have been described. The increase in coronary heart disease, lung cancer and traffic accidents in Europe and North America during the past few decades are examples of modern slow epidemics of non-communicable diseases. Increasing use of drugs has brought epidemics due to their untoward effects, for example phocomelia due to thalidomide. The proliferation of new therapeutic agents makes it likely that such epidemics will be a continuing problem, and doctors have a special responsibility in their early detection and control.

A number of large-scale epidemics have arisen from chemical contamination of food. Outbreaks of organic mercury poisoning, with resulting deaths and neurological disability, have occurred in several countries as a result of ingestion of wheat treated with methyl and ethyl mercury compounds. This wheat was intended only for use as seed, and warnings that it had been treated with mercury to prevent fungus infection and was therefore unfit to eat were not understood by farmers.

New diseases

From time to time there are epidemics of hitherto unrecognized diseases. The first recognized cases of AIDS occurred in the USA in 1981. The earliest indication was an outbreak of *Pneumocystis carinii* pneumonia in young men. This was detected by routine surveillance of cases of pneumonia, by cause, at the Centers of Disease Control — a dramatic example of the worth of routine surveillance of infective disease. Further inquiry showed the cases to be young men who were both homosexual and immunocompromised. The virus was discovered in 1983.

INVESTIGATING AN INFECTIOUS DISEASE EPIDEMIC

In the investigation of an infectious disease epidemic it is wise to follow a systematic routine, even though public reaction, urgency and the local situation may make this difficult. The following list of steps need not always be undertaken in the order given; some are done concurrently. The routine is also a model for investigating non-infectious disease epidemics.

1. Verification of the diagnosis.
2. Confirmation of the existence of an epidemic.
3. Identification of affected persons and their characteristics.
   a. Case histories.
   b. Search for additional cases.
4. Definition and investigation of the population at risk.
5. Formulation of a hypothesis as to source and spread of epidemic.
6. Management of the epidemic.
   a. Treatment of cases.
   b. Prevention of spread and commencement of control measures.
   c. Writing a report.
   d. Continued surveillance of the population.
7. Experimental verification of agent of disease and mode of spread.

Verification of the diagnosis

In developing countries the initial notification of an epidemic is often made by an auxiliary. When an epidemic is notified as detailed a history as possible should be taken from the informants. If the information was received by telegram from a rural district then a radio call back to the nearest police station may elicit more details. A tentative differential diagnosis may then be made, for example 'food poisoning or cholera', 'encephalitis or meningitis'; this enables the doctor to anticipate what diagnostic specimens may be required and what kind of equipment, such as microscope, slides, containers, culture media or lumbar puncture sets, should be taken to the outbreak. The laboratory which will process the specimens can be alerted, and may have to make special arangements such as meeting transport from the epidemic area at awkward hours of the day or night.

With some diseases, such as Lassa fever, the urgency of the situation demands that immediate action is taken on the basis of a clinical diagnosis alone, although laboratory confirmation must be obtained subsequently. For most diseases there is less urgency and a doctor called to an outbreak of typhoid is incautious if he begins collecting information about food and water supplies before verifying that the diagnosis of typhoid is in fact correct.

In some epidemics it is necessary to confirm the diagnosis on cases who have died, and the extent of the autopsy required must be considered. In certain circumstances a complete autopsy is unnecessary (or will antagonize the population who will then conceal deaths), and only limited specimens such as viscerotomy specimens (yellow fever) or rectal swabs (cholera) need be taken.

Confirmation of the existence of an epidemic

Sometimes doctors suddenly start to diagnose a disease which, although previously present in an area, was unrecognized; or new treatment attracts to clinics and hospitals people who previously had relied on traditional medicines. Increase in ascertainment may thus give a false impression of an epidemic, and when investigating an epidemic it is necessary to obtain an approximate estimate of previous incidence of the disease, both from clinic and hospital data and by questioning the local people.

The existence of the epidemic should be demonstrated by a graph of incidence against time and by mapping its geographic extent. When the graph is constructed the time scale should not commence at the epidemic period but should begin at the earliest time for which data are available. When a disease is endemic an epidemic is said to have begun when the incidence rises above a normal endemic level. Various indices of endemicity may be used according to whether or not the disease has a cyclic pattern of occurrence. For diseases showing seasonal variations the mean may be taken of incidence rates for particular weeks or months over the previous several years, or mean high and low levels over a period of years may be calculated.

A simple method of mapping is to use pins, each pin representing a case, with different colours to show different days or weeks of onset. The charting of movement of an epidemic is important, as it facilitates the swift application of control measures to newly affected areas.

Identification of affected persons and their characteristics

Case histories

Details of each confirmed or suspected case must be taken in order to obtain a complete picture of the epidemic. The usual details required are name, age, sex, occupation, place of residence, recent movements, details of symptoms (including time of onset), and dates of previous immunization. Other details taken will depend on what is suspected. For example, if the epidemic seems likely to have arisen from food poisoning then exact details of what has been eaten are required.

For contagious disorders lists of possible source contacts at the time of infection may be required, if the *incubation period* is known. (The incubation period may be defined as the time between infection with the disease agent and the first appearance of signs or symptoms attributable to the disease.) These contacts will have to be interviewed and investigated. Similarly lists of all contacts who could have been infected by the patient will be required.

All this information is best recorded on specially prepared record forms. If large numbers of cases (more than about a thousand) are involved the data will require coding and analysis by computer. A preliminary form must be worked out and duplicated either before departing for the site of the epidemic or at the site. (Often a local school will have a duplicating machine and typewriter, but is unlikely to have sufficient stencils and other stationery.)

Search for additional cases

Initial notification of an epidemic may come from a hospital, but visits to health centres and dispensaries in the area, and further inquiry in the villages, may reveal many cases that were never hospitalized or perhaps were deliberately concealed. Sometimes apparently dissimilar cases prove to be different forms of the same disease. For such reasons the extent of many epidemics is not clearly defined at first. Only the ears of the hippopotamus are visible but the bulk lies below the surface of water!

Definition and investigation of the population at risk

Analysis of the case histories will give a profile in terms of age, sex, place of residence etc. of those affected by the disease. In order to give an epidemiological description of the outbreak this profile must be related to the characteristics and distribution of the entire population at risk. Although available population data may be limited an attempt should be made to calculate attack rates in each area being investigated. The *attack rate* relates the number of cases to the population at risk, and whenever possible age/sex-specific attracts rates should be calculated. If a point-source epidemic is suspected the characteristics of the cases must be compared with those of people seemingly exposed but not affected.

Comparison of the cases with a sample of the population at risk may pinpoint a certain experience which is common to the cases but not shared by those not affected by the disease. This could be eating a particular dish, cooking with a particular ingredient, drawing water from one well, or visiting a certain sick person. Having identified one likely experience it is wise to check it again by asking more specific questions. It may be found that someone who apparently shared the common experience of drawing water from a certain well did not get the disease because he always boiled his water. Someone else who got the disease but is not recorded as using the well may have omitted to mention when first questioned that, although he used another well most of the time, he used the suspect well on occasions.

Investigation of the population at risk may require laboratory tests. Carriers are involved in epidemics of meningococcal meningitis or in some outbreaks of cholera, and laboratory investigations are required to identify this link in the chain of infection. Whenever possible organisms should be typed and their sensitivity to chemotherapy determined, so that vaccine or chemoprophylaxis will be appropriate. Serological testing may be necessary to determine patterns of immunity in the population. Additional or previous cases in animals may have to be identified by serological means: the monkey is an important link in the epidemiology of yellow fever in tropical Africa and America.

Formulation of a hypothesis as to source and spread of epidemic

The investigating doctor wishes to know why the epidemic occurred when it did and how the stage came to be set for its occurrence.

Wherever possible the relevant conditions before the epidemic should be determined, in order to assess the crucial influences that, when altered, made the epidemic possible. In dry months human movement may be increased and markets flourish and the spread of diseases such as meningococcal meningitis and influenza may be facilitated. At other times seasonal changes in the temperature and humidity at night facilitate transmission of respiratory organisms among persons sleeping in the same room. Water supplies may change and it is often necessary to have these mapped out and sampled bacteriologically or chemically. Food supplies or housing and sanitation may have to be investigated and a local health inspector or auxiliary, who already has some knowledge of the area, is a useful person to have on the investigation team. If a vector-borne disease is being investigated it may be necessary to bring in specialists to study the life cycles and population dynamics of the insect and animal reservoirs.

If a single cause such as a staphylococcal toxin is postulated for an epidemic of food poisoning it is necessary to determine the source (e.g. an infected lesion on the cook's thumb), the vehicle (e.g. a particular dish), the predisposing circumstances (e.g. a long interval in warm surroundings before consumption) and the portal of entry (the gastrointestinal tract). If an epidemic is multifocal such a detailed reconstruction of the events may be impossible.

All the links in an infectious process must be considered:

1. The agent of disease and its characteristics
2. The reservoir (man as a case or carrier, other mammals, insects, birds, reptiles, inanimate objects, plants, water or soil)
3. The mode of exit from this reservoir or source
4. The mode of transmission to the next host
5. The mode of entry
6. The susceptibility of the host

Management of the epidemic

Treatment of cases

The doctor who investigates an epidemic must also assume responsibility for treatment of the cases he diagnoses. In an epidemic of meningitis, plague, or cholera emergency accommodation may have to be found and additional staff may have to be given essential training very rapidly. Health auxiliaries, medical students, or even the army may be available for this. For epidemic diseases such as sleeping sickness and cholera treatment is specialized, and may need drugs and equipment not usually found in rural hospitals. It may fall on the investigating doctor to make estimates of requirements and obtain such supplies urgently. Diseases such as poliomyelitis leave in their wake many patients with an immediate need for physiotherapy and rehabilitation; timely organization of these services will lessen the aftermath of deformities.

Prevention of spread and commencement of control measures

Once the epidemiology of the outbreak has been elucidated it is possible to plan a complete control programme. However, even at the onset of his investigations the doctor must attempt to limit spread and the occurrence of new cases.

Many communicable diseases can be prevented by chemoprophylaxis or immunization. Plague and malaria are examples of the first and poliomyelitis and measles of the second. For meningococcal meningitis the type of organism and its sensitivity dictate the applicability of either vaccine or chemoprophylaxis. In addition to chemoprophylaxis and immunization other immediate control measures may be isolation of affected individuals and the imposition of quarantine to prevent movement in or out of an area.

Whatever the urgency for commencement of vaccination or other measures time must also be found to explain the situation to the community at risk and to ensure their co-operation. People's willingness to do such things as report new cases, attend for vaccination or improve standards of hygiene are often critical factors in epidemic control.

Frequently sufficient vaccine or chemoprophylactic agents is not immediately available, and it becomes necessary to define the groups within the community who need priority in the allocation of available supplies. During a recent epidemic of poliomyelitis analysis of the case histories showed that 90% of those affected were under 4 years old. This age-group was made the main target for immunization and it was estimated that 84 000 doses of vaccine would be needed. Only a few thousand were available. Epidemiological analysis of the cases showed that attack rates were seven times higher in villages largely composed of recent migrants into the area than in established villages. Accordingly the available vaccine was allocated to the children under 4 years old living in these villages.

After immediate control measures have been put into action it may be necessary to initiate more permanent ones, which may include improvement of personal hygiene through health education, provision of better water supplies, control of vector breeding or killing of vectors, and food hygiene legislation and enforcement. Long-term plans for continued vaccination after an initial mass programme may also be required.

Writing a report

It is usual to write reports after investigation of an epidemic. These may be for three kinds of reader: first, a popular account for laypeople so that they understand the nature of the epidemic and what is required of them to prevent spread or recurrence; second, an account for planners in the Ministry of Health or local authority so as to ensure that all the necessary administrative steps are taken to limit the outbreak or prevent recurrence; and third, a scientific report for publication in a medical journal. Reports of recent epidemics are invaluable aids when teaching medical staff or auxiliaries about epidemic control.

Continued surveillance of the population

During the acute phase of an epidemic it is necessary to keep the individuals at special risk (e.g. contacts) under surveillance. After the epidemic is under control it becomes necessary to keep the community under surveillance to detect further rises in incidence and to ensure the effectiveness of the selected control measures. The best surveillance method is that which keeps all links of the chain (infectious agent, reservoir, route of transmission and levels of immunity) under close scrutiny. Early detection of a recurrence of the epidemic will enable it to be limited to the smallest number of victims.

The sources of information which can be utilized for surveillance are firstly, notifications of illness by medical staff, auxiliaries, chiefs, employers of labour, schoolteachers, heads of families; secondly, certification of deaths by medical authorities; and thirdly, data from other sources such as public health laboratories, entomological and veterinary services. It may be necessary to maintain a continuous check on the immune status of the population by relating the amount of vaccine used to the estimated number of births. Reporting from the sources listed may be inadequate and a special surveillance team may be needed while the threat continues. Staff engaged in surveillance are trained in the early accurate recognition of the disease, or in identification of the causative agent.

Experimental verification of agent of disease and mode of spread

Occasionally experimental evidence is needed to verify hypotheses about an epidemic. For example, it may be necessary to show that sliced meat can be contaminated by an infected slicing machine, or that tin cans can be infected after canning if they have small holes in them. Such investigations usually require more laboratory facilities than are available in the field, and are often not completed until long after the epidemic has been controlled.

10. Trials of preventive measures

One of the purposes of epidemiology, as stated in Chapter 1, is the evaluation of methods used to control disease. There are two stages in the evaluation of control measures. Firstly a *trial* of the measure is carried out on an 'experimental' population, to determine whether its application to the general population is merited. Secondly the measure is applied to the general population with continuing observation to ensure its efficacy.

As well as evaluating methods to control disease, trials are sometimes used to test hypotheses which arise from observational epidemiology. Associations found in observational studies are influenced by many confounding variables, some of which the investigator may not know. Randomized trials, whose aim is to reduce the effect of confounding variables, will clarify whether associations are causal.

For example, bednets are commonly used in some areas of West Africa with the aim of preventing malaria. When children who slept under bednets were compared to those who did not they were found to have a lower incidence of malaria. This suggested that bednets were protective. However, in a subsequent preventive trial villages in which bednets were not used were randomized to use nets or not. There was no difference in the incidence of childhood malaria between villages who used the bednets and those who did not, even though people in villages asked to use nets did so. This appears to contradict the observational data. The answer, supported by entomological data, seems to be that children who sleep near to users of bednets have an increased number of infective bites, and therefore bednets divert mosquitoes to other children more strongly than they protect the children beneath them.

Measures taken to prevent disease are sometimes classified as primary, secondary or tertiary, according to the stage in disease natural history at which they act. Primary prevention is effective in the early stages of pathogenesis, when an agent of disease (e.g. a parasite) or an environmental influence (e.g. a carcinogen) interacts with a person. Examples of primary preventive measures include vector control, immunization, and environmental sanitation. Once the interaction of agent, environment and person has occurred, secondary preventive measures are required to forestall the occurrence or at least the progression of the illness beyond the acute stage. These measures comprise early diagnosis (e.g. by screening, case-finding) and prompt treatment. Tertiary prevention acts to arrest the course of an illness, once established, and the measures include convalescent care and rehabilitation.

This classification of preventive measures is useful in that it shows the artificial division between preventive and curative or therapeutic medicine, and emphasizes the responsibility of doctors to prevent progression of disease at all stages in the natural history. However in general usage disease prevention is synonymous with primary prevention, and in this chapter the term 'preventive trials' is used to describe trials of primary preventive measures. In part the methodology is similar to that of clinical trials.

A trial of the effect of BCG vaccination on tuberculosis provides a suitable example for discussion. The intention of such a trial is to determine whether or not the large-scale administration of BCG should be selected as a method of TB control in the area being studied. An *experimental population* is chosen from what may be termed the *reference population*, which is the entire population who would be given BCG if the results of the trial were sufficiently encouraging. A reference population may be the population of part of a country, or many countries. The experimental population is divided into a study group, who receive BCG, and a control group, who do not, and the occurrence of tuberculosis in the two groups is compared. The full assessment of BCG as a preventive measure depends upon:

1. its *effectiveness* as indicated by the comparative morbidity and mortality from TB in the vaccinated and unvaccinated groups
2. its *cost* in terms of money and manpower and consequently the feasibility of using it on a large scale
3. any *risks* consequent upon its use.

Clearly a decision to carry out a preventive trial involves important ethical considerations. Exposure of the study group to the possible hazards of the trial can only be justified by the benefits which a successful outcome to the trial may confer on the reference population.

Use of a control group may also raise ethical issues. In a trial of measles vaccine, for example, the investigator may have good evidence at the outset of the trial that the vaccine confers some degree of protection. In order to quantify the degree of protection by means of a trial it is necessary to delay vaccinating the control group.

One cannot impose a trial on a community which does not wish for it, and throughout a trial the experimental population must be informed of the purposes of the trial and any hazards to which they may be liable. In trials carried out on children the permission of the parents is, of course, necessary. Although schools may seem to provide convenient populations for preventive trials the difficulties of communication with parents, who may reside far from the school, can make their use impracticable.

The design of a preventive trial may be considered under the sequence of headings given in Chapters 3 to 8.

Choosing a population

The factors governing choice of the experimental population, on whom the trial will be carried out, may be considered under three headings.

1. It must be *representative* of the reference population. Experimental populations are usually communities living in a defined area. Practical considerations usually make it impossible to draw random, and therefore theoretically representative, samples from the reference population. The administration of a preventive trial requires experimental populations to be geographically grouped so that the individuals in the trial can be readily observed. However, while admitting that the experimental population will not be truly representative, it is essential that it should be as representative of the reference population as is feasible. It would be inappropriate to carry out a BCG trial in a country on groups of refugees living there. Although choice of a refugee settlement may facilitate the administrative problems of a trial, the refugees' previous experience of tuberculosis and their population structure in respect of age and other variables is likely to be quite unrepresentative of the general population among whom they live. It would therefore be impossible

to use the results of a BCG trial on refugees to predict the effectiveness of BCG in the country as a whole.

2. The *incidence* of the disease in the experimental population should correspond to that in the reference population. As is discussed later in this chapter, the size of the experimental population is determined by the numbers of cases of the disease which are required to demonstrate differences in disease rates in the control and study groups. If there is a high incidence of the disease in the experimental population the size of the population required will be smaller than if the incidence is low. However, the influences which determine a high incidence of a disease in a community may also make the response to a preventive measure atypical of the reference population. Unless there is evidence to show that this objection to the use of a high-incidence community cannot be sustained, then it will be preferable to select a community in which the incidence is around the mean for the reference population.

3. The experimental population must be suitable to the *practical requirements* of a preventive trial. The population must have similar characteristics to those required in cohort studies. It must be available for the duration of the trial, i.e. not liable to substantial migrations; co-operative and likely to remain so throughout the trial; and easily accessible to the investigators so that the expense and labour of the trial are minimized. There is often a wide choice of experimental populations open to the investigator, and no one will knowingly choose a nomadic community hostile towards modern medicine when a settled community with more progressive views will serve the same purpose.

Size of the experimental population

In Chapter 3 a brief account is given of the way in which sample size is related to the statistical precision with which rates, or the mean values of quantitative variables, observed in samples reflect the true rates or means in the parent population. In general the larger the sample the greater the precision. In preventive trials the investigator is making simultaneous observations on at least two samples, the study group and the control group. In each group a disease rate or the values of a quantitative variable are recorded and comparison is then made between the two. Since the rates or values recorded in each sample are inexact estimates of the rates or values in the population, it follows that the comparison between the two groups is likewise inexact.

In a BCG trial comparison is made of the difference between the tuberculosis rates in the study group, given BCG, and the unvaccinated control group. The precision of this difference depends upon the magnitude of the difference and the size of the two samples. Therefore when designing the trial the investigator specifies the minimum reduction which would make BCG a useful preventive measure for the reference population. He then specifies an acceptable range of error for the difference. These two considerations, coupled with the incidence of the disease in the control group, will enable calculation of the required sample size.

Having decided on the sample size, let us say 5000 individuals in the study group and the same number in the control group, it is necessary to allow for the non-co-operation of a proportion of individuals in the two groups. If it is predicted that 10% of the individuals will either fail to co-operate from the outset or will become unavailable during the course of the trial an additional 500 individuals will be required in each group. Similarly other causes of loss to follow-up must be allowed for. If the BCG were to be given to neonates in a country with high infant mortality the sample size would need to be increased accordingly. The unpredictability of the effects of the AIDS epidemic on adult mortality has made this point particularly important and difficult.

The choice of the outcome measure itself also influences sample size. If overall mortality were to be the end-point then the trial would need to be considerably larger as tuberculosis contributes a relatively small fraction of deaths. This point becomes philosophical to some extent, and indeed controversial, but it is feasible that an intervention might reduce mild disease, or its measurable impact, whilst not influencing severe and fatal disease.

The foregoing is a brief account of the reasoning which determines the size of the experimental population. In practice there are many administrative considerations which influence the final choice of the population, and an investigator without previous experience would be unwise to specify the population without prior discussion with an epidemiologist or statistician familiar with the problem.

Selection of controls

For most kinds of preventive trial it is essential that part of the experimental population is used as a control group. Although it may simplify the administration of a trial if there is no control group, and the incidence of the disease in the experimental population after exposure to the preventive measure is compared with that in the period preceding exposure, this is rarely a satisfactory procedure. Secular changes in the incidence of diseases are common, and a decline in incidence during the course of a trial may be quite unrelated to the preventive measure being tested.

It may be argued that in the past the effectiveness of a number of preventive measures was demonstrated without the use of control groups. With the issue of fruit juice to sailors scurvy ceased to be a hazard of long sea voyages. More recent was the dramatic and almost complete disappearance of paralytic poliomyelitis in many countries following the introduction of Salk (later Sabin) vaccine. However the circumstances of such successes were special in several respects. Firstly, the effect of the preventive measures was unusually large and rapid. Secondly, they were widely adopted over a short period of time. Thirdly, there were no other changes which could have accounted for the swift decline in disease. Lastly, the incidence of the disease had been adequately documented before the preventive measure was introduced.

Although paralytic poliomyelitis has almost disappeared in many countries it recently reappeared in Oman and The Gambia, two countries with high vaccination rates. It seems that seroconversion does not always follow vaccination in developing countries. Controlled trials of polio vaccine are now needed to determine which vaccine regimes give the higher seroconversion.

Comparison of disease incidence in a study group with that in a control group is, in most circumstances, the only sure method of measuring the effectiveness of a preventive measure. Therefore when the experimental population has been defined it is first subdivided into study and control groups. It is convenient to restrict discussion of the procedures for making the subdivision to an example where there is one study group and one control group. In practice there may be a number of study groups each of which, for example, receives a different dose of vaccine. Such trials will require a more complex sample size calculation but the procedures for selecting multiple study or control groups are basically the same as those used for single groups.

The problems associated with selection of controls in preventive trials differ from those in analytic studies, described in Chapter 4. In analytic studies a group of patients or a study cohort is defined and a control group or cohort is sought from some other source.

In trials the experimental population is the source of both the study and control groups. Allocation of individuals to either group must conform as far as possible to the ideals of random selection so that if, to take the simplest example, the study and control groups are to be of equal size each individual must have an equal likelihood of allocation to one or other group.

The procedures which may be used are as follows:

1. Random sampling
2. Community randomization
3. Stratified sampling.

Random sampling

If the experimental population has been listed before the trial, for example when a BCG trial is preceded by Mantoux testing, individuals may be allocated to the study and control groups by use of random numbers. The allocation of each individual to the vaccinated or unvaccinated group is therefore known before vaccination is begun. Allocation of individuals cannot be made from a list of 'possible' participants; it can only be done from a list of those who have been consulted and have agreed to participate. Frequently it is impracticable to obtain a preliminary listing of participants and their identity is unknown until their attendance at the beginning of the trial. In this event one of two procedures may be used. Each individual may be given a number corresponding to the order of his attendance, and each of these numbers is randomly allocated to the study or control group beforehand. Alternatively, in trials in which a placebo is given the vials of vaccine and placebo can be placed in a random order and allocated to individuals in the order they attend.

When the experimental population is followed up it is preferable that neither the members of the population nor the trial staff responsible for follow-up are aware of which people belong to the study group and which to the control. This ensures that there is no bias which, for example, can result if individuals, knowing that they are controls, become less willing to co-operate than the study individuals, or if the trial staff give more interest and attention to the study than the control group. It also prevents manipulation of the random allocation at clinics to ensure that friends get the active (supposedly better) intervention. A trial in which the experimental population is unaware of who is a study or control individual is called a *blind trial*. If the trial staff responsible for follow-up are also unaware then the trial is *double-blind*. Simple techniques may be used to ensure that the trial staff are unaware of the identity of the individuals they observe. In a recent BCG trial the arms of all participants were covered by a sticking plaster at the site where the BCG was injected or, for the control group, would have been injected had they received it. The staff therefore could not observe the presence or absence of a BCG scar.

Random sampling of the experimental population by the methods described ensures that the identity of the study and control groups is known only to those members of the trial staff who have access to the original records. Systematic sampling, which may be used for selection of controls in analytic studies, is inappropriate to preventive trials. A system such as alternate allocation of individuals to one or other group in order of their initial attendance is likely to reveal the identity of the groups to the trial staff and may also be comprehended by the participants.

Community randomization

Although random sampling of individuals is the ideal statistical procedure it is not always feasible. Some preventive measures are applied to communities rather than to individuals. A trial of the efficacy of molluscicides in controlling bilharzia requires comparison of a community in an area where the water is treated with a community in an area where the water is untreated. In trials of this kind it is important to choose study and control communities which are as similar as possible with respect of all factors that are likely to influence incidence of the disease. It is an inherent flaw in the design of such trials that the two communities are nevertheless likely to be dissimilar in some respects, and that a fluctuation in disease incidence unrelated to the preventive measure may occur in one or other of them during the course of the trial. For example, there may be a sharp rise in incidence of bilharzia in one community resulting from breakage of a borehole pump and consequent necessity of using a nearby river as a domestic water-source, while the incidence in the adjacent community remains unchanged. Such local changes of incidence may result in under- or over-estimation of the effect of the preventive measure. The investigator must be aware of this possibility and can to some extent guard against it by choosing more than one study and control community. The number of communities needed in such trials is not easily estimated but one essential piece of information will be the variation in the outcome measure, e.g. bilharzia rates, from village to village. These data will usually have to be collected in a pilot study. Analysis of trials of this type is not straightforward and it is best to work with statisticians familiar with the design problems.

Stratified sampling

As in cohort studies the study and control groups in a trial must be comparable with respect to the distribution of variables and attributes which influence the frequency of the disease. Random allocation of individuals to the study or control groups is carried out in order to achieve this comparability. But the chance factors which operate in a random sampling procedure may sometimes result in the distributions of age, for example, being dissimilar in the two groups. This is less likely to occur when the groups are large, and if recognized at the time of analysis can be allowed for. But the likelihood of its occurrence can be minimized if the experimental population is stratified into age-groups, and individuals in each age-group are randomly allocated, in the correct proportion, to the study and control groups. The need for stratification is greatest when the frequency of the disease being studied shows marked variations, with age, sex, or some other variable or attribute, and when the experimental population is small.

Stratification of communities can also be done if these are the units of the trial and, in this way, village-to-village variation can be adjusted for. For example, in a study of chemoprophylaxis against malaria where the village health worker dispenses the tablets the unit of randomization must clearly be villages. However one might carry out a pilot study to determine spleen size in the children in the villages and stratify the randomization of villages by their average enlarged spleen rate.

Record design

In designing records for preventive trials particular attention may be needed to ensure that observations made on any individual during the trial can be related to previous observations on that individual. This is the problem of record linkage, and its solution depends on two requirements being met. First each individual must have an unique identification, so that observations made on him or her are unerringly related to one individual and the investigator is not faced with the dilemma of deciding which of three adult women named Kandole has a positive sputum report. Usually the combination of name, age, sex, parents' names, birthplace and address provides sufficient identification, but it may also be helpful if each individual is given a small card covered with polythene which shows the trial number and other identification data. If each participant keeps his identity card and shows it at follow-up interviews or examinations his record card may be more easily located. It will still be necessary to check that this is indeed the correct individual as cards may be exchanged or mixed up in the family.

The second requirement for manual record linkage is that the records are ordered in a way that enables swift recovery of a participant's record once the identification data are known. Records may be grouped under families within villages, or they may be ordered according to the sequence of trial numbers, with provision of a register to enable the trial number of those who lose their identity cards to be determined. Any system of filing the records is suitable so long as it works. Although computers greatly simplify linkage, a manual system of recording may still be needed in the field. In both computerized and field records it will be necessary to ensure that the observer cannot gain access to the code that determines which intervention the subject received.

The general principles of record design described in Chapter 6 apply to trial records in the same way as to other types of epidemiological records.

Fieldwork techniques

A BCG trial may require observation of the experimental population for up to 5 or more years, and throughout this time the cooperation and interest of the population must be maintained. One method of ascertaining cases of tuberculosis in the population will be to have regular clinics in the area, to which people with coughs or other symptoms may report. If they are properly informed about the nature of the disease and the availability of treatment it is likely that they will avail themselves of the facilities offered at the clinic. If they receive treatment from which they perceive a benefit this will benefit the community even if the trial is negative. Treatment, however, may reduce the incidence of the disease under study and so reduce the statistical power of the study. (This is especially true if the major outcome is death.) On the other hand it may facilitate detection of disease and increase the incidence. So that bias is not introduced the treatment facility must be equally accessible to study and control groups.

It may be necessary to have an initial survey of the entire experimental population to detect all existing cases of TB, since the inclusion of cases of TB in the study or control groups at the beginning of the trial will prejudice the precision with which the trial measures the effectiveness of the vaccine. During the trial an aڂernative to ascertainment of TB through regular clinics is periodic reviews of the population. Although this may be time-consuming and costly it is likely to give a higher level of case detection than the clinics, and may thereby enable the trial to be completed in less time. Shortening of the trial may effect a saving in money and manpower which more than compensates for the cost and effort required for periodic resurveys. A combination of methods may be used to maximize information. In trials of malaria prevention a pre-intervention survey for prevalence of parasitaemia anaemia and splenomegaly is carried out. After the intervention there is continuous monitoring of episodes of malaria in the population and a final cross-sectional survey of the initial parameters.

The application of certain preventive measures depends upon the active involvement of the population. Changes is eating, smoking, drinking or agricultural practices require a more intense relationship with a community than vaccination does. It is generally found that preventive measures which require behavioural change are less successful than those such as vaccination or insecticide spraying, which require only consent. Continued active participation usually depends on a mechanism of frequent encouragement and reinforcement.

Analysis

The crucial result of a trial is the demonstration of whether or not disease incidence in the study group is lower than that in the control group. It is not sufficient to show that a particular measure improves the results of laboratory tests: the measures of outcome should be those which are directly important to the subjects, that is to say death, disability or symptoms. However, *criteria of effectiveness* will include other comparisons between the groups, for example of the severity and age distribution of the disease. Analysis should also include an assessment of any risks to the recipients of the preventive measure, e.g. encephalopathy following whooping cough vaccination, and estimation of the money and manpower costs of large-scale application of the preventive measure. For the latter the assistance of a health economist will usually be required. It may be difficult to separate the research costs of the trial from the intervention costs if this is not considered in the design stage. As so few trials of public health measures are carried out it is important that the intervention tested is as similar as possible to that which would be introduced by the government. This ensures that the trial results are directly applicable to public health practice.

Before comparing the disease patterns in the two groups it is necessary to consider two points.

First, are the two groups comparable in terms of the distribution of age, sex and other variables or attributes which are related to the incidence of the disease? The procedure used to divide the experimental population into study and control groups may have failed to achieve adequate similarity between them, or there may have been different patterns of non-co-operation and migration so that the eventual composition of the two groups of participants is dissimilar. If there are important dissimilarities the incidence of the disease in each group may be standardized to allow for them (see Ch. 8).

Secondly, what proportion of the participants failed to conform to the study and control programmes? If the follow-up rate in the two groups is very different this may bias the result. If subjects in the control group received the active measure elsewhere or subjects in the study group got repeat vaccinations the analysis must ignore this.

In a trial of a preventive measure which requires the continued participation of the experimental population, such as use of a new borehole as a domestic water source, it is likely that part of the study group will change their mind and not alter their behaviour. For reasons of convenience or preference they may revert to old customs of fetching water from nearby rivers, lakes, or swamps. It may seem that the effectiveness of the preventive measure should be assessed from the disease occurrence among only those who complied with the programme. However, such an assessment represents a potential effectiveness rather than a realizable one, for in any population there are likely to be people who do not comply. The correct assessment of the effectiveness of the measure is therefore one which includes these people. If a trial fails to show that the measure is effective it is important to identify non-compliance as a possible source of failure. If compliance was poor then the measure should not be finally abandoned until methods of achieving better compliance have been explored; but in the meantime it should not, of course, be implemented in the reference population.

Analysis of a preventive trial must result in a clear statement about the benefit the community will derive from the measure; the risks; and the costs in terms of money and manpower if the measure is adopted. Final decisions to apply preventive measures on a large scale are usually made by politicians and non-medical administrators, and their medical advisers are expected to present them with a clear and succinct summary of the benefits and disadvantages of each method being considered.

11. Evaluation of health services

This chapter describes some of the many kinds of information which may be collected in order to measure the health needs of a community and implement appropriate services. Such information is obviously essential to health workers occupying posts which carry with them a defined responsibility for the health of a community, for example District Medical Officers and nurses in charge of maternity and child health. But those appointed to work solely within hospitals or clinics should also collect epidemiological data about their patients. A surgeon who finds that he is spending many hours a month skin-grafting children with burns will wish to find out why so many children in his area are being burnt, and what simple measures could prevent it. A paediatrician with a ward full of children with advanced kwashiorkor will think about the means for effecting earlier diagnosis and prevention, and will wish for a numerical assessment of the nutritional problems in the area. A nurse seeing many babies with neonatal tetanus will want information about home delivery practices in the area.

RECORDS

Health workers seeking answers to particular questions will usually have to collect the data themselves. Sometimes these data will be available from routine records, of which there are three types in most developing countries — censuses, hospitals and clinics.

Census data

Census data are used to determine the size of populations at risk. Rural-to-urban migration is now so frequent in many countries, and birth rates are so high, that the data may need to be adjusted within 2 or 3 years of the census. In small areas migration may introduce such large errors that a special census may be necessary before a health survey is undertaken. During a census the enumeration of some population groups, such as people in urban slums, or children in the first year of life, is often incomplete. It is wise to consult someone with detailed knowledge of the particular census before using the data.

Routine data on births and deaths are available in some countries, but must be interpreted with caution. Many births occur at home and are not registered, or are registered late; cause of death is often not accurate.

Hospital data

Hospitals and clinics provide the most readily available information about disease in a community. Hospital inpatient data will be the most diagnostically accurate, because clinical diagnoses will be supported by laboratory investigations; these data tell one whether diseases such as kala-azar and meningococcal meningitis occur in a community.

However, there are two usual limitations to the usefulness of information obtained from these sources. Firstly, only a minority of the population may use hospital services, and the pattern of disease among people requesting treatment is usually unrepresentative of the pattern in the community. Morbidity rates derived from them will therefore be biased. This does not render them worthless, for at the least they will reveal some of the common diseases in the area and may highlight sections of the community who are at high risk of disease and for whom special services are necessary. Furthermore if the bias remains approximately constant, in that there is no major change in the provision or use of health services in the area, then information from hospitals may be used to monitor the changing frequency of disease and give early warning of epidemics. An example would be fluctuations in the numbers of cases of meningococcal meningitis.

The second limitation is that record-keeping is often incomplete, or even non-existent. The quality of records must be assessed before any analysis of them is carried out. It may be found that staff have not been properly trained in keeping records. Certain diagnostic categories may be unreliable — for example, all cases of fever may be recorded as malaria. The records may fail to distinguish first attendances and subsequent attendances for the same complaint. Occasionally there may be over-reporting, to justify requests for additional staff or drugs. The quality of records can often be improved inexpensively by training or motivating existing staff or providing an additional clerk. A key group for motivation is the doctors. They will often not keep records because they are too busy and because they do not appreciate the usefulness of relatively simple data. Feedback of results and demonstration of the resultant action will often be the best stimulus to better records.

Clinic data

Records of patients attending health centres and maternal and child health clinics are often kept routinely. Their quality, however, varies and partly depends on the motivation of the staff who complete them. Difficulties arise when the statistics produced are only used centrally, and are of no immediate relevance to the staff or the community that they serve. This can be overcome by feeding results of analyses that are relevant to their work back to the staff or, even better, by training the staff to analyse and apply their own statistics. A health inspector responsible for recording cases of immunizable diseases, and for vaccinating children, will see the relevance of geographical patterns of measles in his area more easily than someone sitting in an office many hundreds of kilometres away. If in addition it is he who goes and investigates outbreaks, record-keeping becomes of interest to him.

Intensive data collection on a number of diseases or specific, highly detailed information on one disease is best done in selected areas only. This underlies the concept of *sentinel reporting units*. Here staff are especially trained to recognize particular diseases of interest and may be given additional diagnostic tools. An accurate census of the population at risk will allow rates of disease to be calculated. Sentinel surveillance is especially appropriate for unusual diseases or diseases with strong epidemicity or seasonality. If the sentinel units are chosen appropriately, as representative of the population both from the point of view of geography and high-risk groups, they will give early warning of epidemics or failings of the routine services.

SPECIAL SURVEYS

Depending on the particular problem being investigated the relatively crude information obtained from hospitals and clinics may or may not be sufficient. If it is not, a survey will be needed; the type of survey required will depend on the questions being asked. Evaluation of nutritional status or vaccine coverage will require a cross-sectional study. Uncommon conditions such as leprosy or paralytic polio will require case-finding. Questions on risk factors for illness will require a case-control study. These three common types of survey will be illustrated by a nutrition survey, a leprosy survey and a case-control study of neonatal tetanus.

A nutrition survey

A cross-sectional study

A nutrition survey illustrates the techniques used for diseases with a high prevalence, other examples of which in many communities would be the major parasitic infestations.

If a doctor finds that numbers of children with protein–calorie malnutrition are attending his clinics a nutrition survey of the community becomes a high priority. For every patient with kwashiorkor there may be 15 others with mild or moderate malnutrition. A preliminary survey of the community will serve to define the extent and causes of the problem, to pinpoint groups in most urgent need, and to show the appropriate methods of control. Although preliminary nutritional assessment of all age-groups within the community may be the ideal, surveys are commonly limited to children under 3 years of age because of their especial vulnerability to malnutrition. Since malnutrition tends to be widespread in communities it is necessary to carry out a sample survey with detailed examination of all young children in the sample.

The essentials of one kind of simple, quick and inexpensive nutrition survey may be considered under five headings:

1. The sample.
2. The record form.
3. Execution of the survey.
4. The analysis.
5. The action.

The sample

Cluster samples will usually be required because of their convenience for the fieldworkers. Where people live in villages or other small groupings these form ready made cluster samples, as described in Chapter 3. But where people's homes are scattered it is necessary for the investigator to define clusters.

Suppose that the survey is to be carried out over 5 days with two clusters comprising 50 children under 3 years to be examined every day. Initially a listing is obtained of the smallest administrative divisions, e.g. wards and subcounties, within the area to be covered by the survey. Each division may have a population of several thousand people. The divisions are numbered and 10 numbers selected from random number tables. These numbers designate the divisions from within which the clusters will be selected. (One division may be the source of more than one cluster.)

The next step is selection of a household as the starting point for each cluster. If there is a listing of all heads of household within the administrative division, e.g. a tax register, the households may be numbered from the listing. If there is no listing each home within the division may be mapped and a number allocated to it. From the numbered households, either on the listing or on the map, one is selected as the basis for each cluster, again using random number tables. As an alternative to lists of all households within a division it may be possible to use lists of leaders of small groups, e.g. chiefs, political leaders. Random selection of one of these leaders may be followed by selection of one household from a map or household list of his group. In these circumstances it is often necessary to examine the children in the leader's household as well as those required for the survey. The results are likely to be biased in relation to the wealth of the community as a whole and should not be used unless the household is actually included in the random sample.

The record form

An individual record form will be completed for each child included in the survey. This will comprise a number of sections, according to the particular requirements of the survey.

1. *Personal identity*, including name, age, sex, father's and mother's name, address and relationship to head of household will be required in any survey, as described in Chapter 6. The problems of determining age are discussed in Chapter 5. Additional information such as father's occupation or mother's educational level may sometimes be relevant. The date of completion of the record and the interviewer's identity must be recorded.

2. *Anthropometric data*, including weight, height, arm circumference, head circumference and number of erupted teeth. Techniques

for these measurements must be standardized, as described in Chapter 2, so that the technique for measurement of arm circumference, for example, must be defined in detail, including position of the arm, site of measurement, method of holding the tape and precision of reading, e.g. to nearest millimetre.

3. *Clinical signs* of protein–calorie malnutrition. These are subject to observer variation (Ch. 2) and the book by Jelliffe, listed in Suggested Further Reading, should be consulted before selection of the signs to be recorded, e.g. hair changes, oedema.

4. *Other diseases.* Since infection and malnutrition are interdependent some information about the child's medical history may be recorded. The temptation to record too much information must be avoided and a single question on the child's health on the previous day may be sufficient.

Execution of the survey

For each cluster the survey begins at the household selected as the starting point. There are a variety of procedures which can be used to select the 50 young children required in each cluster. One such procedure is to complete a record form for each child under 3 years in the starting household (A) and then move to the nearest household (B) similarly recording information on the young children. The next household (C) is the one closest to B. In this way the survey team move from a household to the nearest one, other than one already surveyed or one outside the administrative division. The cluster is completed by the household in which the 50th child is found. Since all children under 3 in any household must be included there may be one or two more than 50 children in the sample when the final household has been surveyed.

The need to train personnel and test techniques is described in Chapter 2, and fieldwork techniques are described in Chapter 7. A 'household' will require careful definition: generally children are regarded as belonging to the household in which they habitually eat and sleep but problems arise when a child divides its life between several households or is temporarily absent, or has lived in the area for a few weeks only. Precise definition of terms before the survey begins is necessary.

A member of the survey team may have to return to each cluster sample on a day following the survey, perhaps to examine children who were temporarily absent or ensure that those identified as being severely malnourished receive medical care.

The analysis

The following examples illustrate the kinds of analyses which may be made. (An account of epidemiological analysis is given in Ch. 8.)

1. Prevalence of severe protein–calorie malnutrition (defined by reference to an accepted classification) by age-group in each cluster and in the total sample, together with the sampling error. Prevalence of individual signs of malnutrition.

2. Distribution of anthropometric measurements by age-group, expressed as appropriate summarizing indices, e.g. mean and standard error. Relation of these distributions to known standards, for example the Harvard standards of weight for height or height for age.

The action

There is little purpose to the survey unless it is made the basis for reasoned action to prevent malnutrition. The action may come through changes in agricultural practices, food supplementation, day-care centres, nutritional surveillance at young child clinics, immunization campaigns, family planning advice. Whatever the action it must be evaluated. As part of this evaluation further cluster samples may be surveyed, or the same clusters resurveyed, to determine what changes in the nutritional status of the community have been effected by the action taken.

Cross-sectional surveys may be extended to include a so-called KAPE survey. In this the respondents are asked about their *K*nowledge, *At*titudes, *P*ractice and *E*xpectations in relation to a health problem. These surveys may be a guide to action. They can also produce surprising results. In one done recently in West Africa, in conjunction with a vaccination coverage survey, less than 10% of mothers knew what any of the vaccinations their children received was for — despite 70% of all the children being fully immunized with seven antigens.

Leprosy survey

A *case-finding study*

Surveys of less common diseases such as leprosy are usually designed as case-finding surveys within a defined population rather than as sample surveys. A medical officer will often wish to combine measurement of prevalence and distribution by means of a case-finding survey, with the initiation of an effective long-term scheme for treatment and control. Therefore this section outlines a leprosy survey combined with reorganization of an outpatient leprosy programme.

The essentials of the survey may be considered under five headings:

1. Case-finding methods
2. The record form
3. Execution of the survey
4. The analysis
5. The action.

Case-finding methods

Suppose that during the survey an attempt will be made to identify all cases of leprosy within a district of 100 000 people. Published data suggest that the prevalence of leprosy will be of the order of 8 per 1000 total population and the survey is therefore expected to identify approximately 800 patients. Only 300 patients are currently registered with the mobile team responsible for district leprosy services.

Successful case-finding depends on good advance publicity and during the weeks preceding the survey medical assistants, nurses, midwives and other health personnel are asked to spend time informing the local people of the purpose of the survey, and the date when it will be carried out in each locality. Twenty locations are selected which the survey team will visit at specified times during one week. Local attitudes to leprosy are explored to determine whether unjustified fear will prevent patients attending for examination, and whether the value of early diagnosis and treatment are understood. In accordance with the suggestions made in Chapter 7 care is taken to ensure co-operation not only from the local population and their leaders, but also from staff at health centres and in the mobile clinic, who may feel that the survey is mounted in criticism of their work. Known leprosy patients are asked to bring their families for examination.

Experience from leprosy surveys in many parts of the world has shown the overwhelming importance of this initial phase whereby the survey is publicized, the support of local leaders of the people obtained, and the people persuaded of the benefits of treatment. Attitudes to leprosy are difficult to change and a survey which does not take sufficient account of the sociological aspects of the disease, the prejudices and customs surrounding it, will fail. A ready test of peoples' genuine interest in the survey may be made by a request for some act of co-operation such as the provision of accommodation for the survey team.

The record form

The survey record can also be used as the continuing clinic record of each patient. Its size and form will be partly determined by the need for storage and repeated access. To withstand repeated handling it will have to be of high-quality card. Before the final form of the record is determined comments from the mobile clinic staff are invited and its use is tried out on a group of patients already attending for treatment. The record is laid out in a number of sections.

1. *Personal identity*. As is usual, the record is headed by personal details of the patient, together with a unique identity number.

2. *Clinical description*. The form lists four major signs of leprosy whose presence or absence must be recorded. The presence of skin infiltration, nodules, or eye signs leads to classification as lepromatous leprosy while hypopigmented anaesthetic skin patches are taken to indicate tuberculoid or other forms. The distribution of skin lesions is recorded on a printed outline drawing of the body. The presence or absence of thickening of five nerves — cervical, ulnar, radial, medial, peroneal — is recorded. The form provides space for notes on the previous history of the patient.

3. *Bacteriology*. The dates on which skin smears are taken, and the results, are recorded.

4. *Health education*. The form lists items of health education about which each patient is informed. For example, exercises for stiff hands and methods for lifting hot cooking pots safely may be demonstrated, and instruction given on the importance of wearing shoes, of daily examination of the hands and feet, of reporting injuries or eye abnormalities early, of taking regular treatment and of attending monthly clinics.

5. *Examination of the family*. Each newly diagnosed patient is asked to bring all members of his or her household for examination at the next clinic attendance, and the results of the examination of

each member are recorded on the card. New patients found in this way are then given a separate card.

6. *Routine assessment*. The results of routine assessment at intervals after the survey are not recorded in free form as is usual in clinical notes, but in pre-coded form (as in Fig. 6.2). Signs of reaction, e.g. tender skin patches or inflamed eyes with reduced vision, together with signs of complications of the disease, e.g. plantar ulcers or burns, are listed on the form and the presence or absence of each is recorded at every attendance. The form states that the presence of any of the listed reactions or complications, excepting burns or injuries, is an indication for referral to the health centre or hospital.

7. *Treatment*. A pre-coded format is used to record details of treatment and the interval before the next visit.

Execution of the survey

During the survey the two main problems will be to ensure the continuing co-operation of the population and to minimize observer variation in the recording of clinical signs of leprosy. At some of the 20 locations visited by the survey team the attendance may be much below that predicted from a leprosy prevalence of 8 per 1000. It will be necessary to spend time finding out the reasons for the low attendance, and members of the team will have to make a second visit to the location on another date. Clinical signs of leprosy such as nerve thickening are known to be subject to observer variation. To minimize this a sample of patients must be examined by more than one observer, so that the observations made by each observer are standardized. (Observer variation is discussed further in Ch. 2.)

The analysis

The results of the survey will give age/sex-specific prevalence rates for leprosy (lepromatous, tuberculoid and other forms). They will show the frequency of different types and degrees of disability, and the proportion of cases who were already attending clinics and taking treatment regularly.

The action

The survey will of itself fulfil several important purposes. It is likely that many new cases will be found; all cases will be examined and classified in a standard way; the treatment of each case will be reviewed; an up-to-date record system will be created which, accompanied by a central register of patients, may be used to ensure that treatment defaulters are swiftly found. The creation of a central register, with duplication of the essential data on each patient, is also a necessary insurance against loss of clinic records. The survey will give health education to patients and encourage those who suspect they have the disease to come forward for treatment. With a well-kept record system the progress of the leprosy programme may be kept under review. Early results may be evident from a reduction in the number of cases progressing to deformity and in the number of treatment defaulters. (A reduction in the number of new cases occurring may not be seen for many years.) The doctor may use periodic reviews of the records as an occasion to show the mobile clinic staff the results of their work and to suggest alterations and improvements.

Cross-sectional and case-finding surveys can be combined. To measure vaccine effectiveness, for example, a cross-sectional survey within a population will estimate how many children at each age have received how many doses of vaccine. A case-finding survey will show the number of doses of vaccine received by each child affected by the disease. Numbers of affected children are related to the number of unaffected children given the same doses of vaccine, and rates of disease by vaccine status are calculated. These rates give a direct measure of vaccine effectiveness. This is a valuable method, particularly in epidemics of immunizable disease, and has been found to give results consistent with those of other measures of vaccine effectiveness, such as the case-control method described below.

Neonatal tetanus

A case-control study

Suppose that a nurse observes an increasing number of newborn children with tetanus and informs the regional health team. After examining the children they confirm that they do indeed have neonatal tetanus, despite the regional policy of antenatal immunization against the disease. They report the problem to the Director of Medical Services who orders an investigation by the Epidemiology Unit. The Unit decide to carry out a case-control study to try to identify the factors that have led to these children becoming infected.

Table 11.1 Questions for diagnosis of neonatal tetanus

Symptoms preceding infant's death (Please circle appropriate answer)		
1. Was the infant able to such milk after birth?	Yes	No
2. Did the infant stop sucking milk when became ill?	Yes	No
3. How many days passed before the infant became ill?	☐	days
4. Did the infant's body become rigid?	Yes	No
5. Did the infant have convulsions?	Yes	No
6. Did the infant have a fever?	Yes	No
7. What does mother say the infant died of? _____		

1. *Definition and selection of cases.* A standardized definition a
case will be necessary. The diagnosis of neonatal tetanus depends
on a child being born alive and developing an illness on the third
day of life or later; during this time there are typical spasms or
convulsions. Table 11.1 gives a standard WHO questionnaire. All
health workers in the region will be asked to report any babies who
may have the disease. These will be reviewed by the survey team
to determine whether or not they satisfy the case definition. Those
born outside the region will be excluded.

2. *Selection of controls.* Three living children from the same village, born within 1 month of the child with tetanus, will be selected. They will be of the same sex as the affected child. The
selection of three control children for every tetanus case will increase the statistical power of the study. Since neonatal tetanus is
seasonal in some places it is important that the controls are born
at the same time of year. The controls should be from the village
and not selected from children attending a health facility; the antenatal and delivery practice of mothers who bring their children
to health centres may differ from those who do not.

3. *Record form.* A form will be completed for each affected child
and control. The respondent to the questions will be the mother of
the child. The form will comprise a number of sections.

   a. *Personal identity,* including name, date of birth and sex of
   the child. There will be a clear indication as to whether this
   is a case or a control, and if a control, to which case he or
   she is matched. The date of the interview will be recorded
   and the name of the interviewer.

   b. *Immunization history* for tetanus will be obtained from every
   mother. Where possible this will be confirmed by reference
   to the antenatal record.

   c. *Details of the delivery* will be recorded and in particular the length of the cord, how it was cut and with what implement, and any application that was put on it. The type of person who attended the delivery will be recorded and where the delivery took place.

4. *Fieldwork*. The team will attempt to visit the mother of the affected child as soon after notification as possible. The record form will be completed at the same time as the medical officer confirms the diagnosis. The controls will be selected by choosing a random direction from the home of the child and then visiting every household in that direction until three suitable controls have been found. The interview will be conducted by the same person for all of the controls and the case in a matched set. The interviewers will all be trained and their work will be supervised by visits at random intervals. The causes of tetanus and how it can be prevented will be explained to all mothers in the study. Those who are not up to date with their tetanus immunization will be re-immunized.

5. *Analysis*. The study will be analysed to determine the protective effectiveness of antenatal tetanus immunization, whether the type of attendant affects the risk of tetanus and whether applications to the cord increase the risk. These will then be considered jointly to see if any risk factor is predominant. A recent study of this sort in Pakistan showed that even if the child was delivered by a physician in hospital the risk of tetanus was not reduced, but there was a large risk associated with application of ghee to the cord. This was done after the child was taken home from hospital.

6. *Action*. This study may lead to important conclusions about the failings of the immunization services or the effects of traditional practices. It could be followed or combined with a survey of mothers' attitudes to determine the best action to be taken. The study described here could be limited in its applicability to the whole population in that it is restricted to children who come to the notice of health workers. It could be combined with a community cross-sectional survey of tetanus deaths. After the study, continued surveillance of tetanus deaths and immunization rates in the community will be necessary.

INTERPRETING DATA

Data collected in surveys will form the basis of public health action. Their interpretation can be considered under three headings — time, place and person.

Time

Changes in disease occurrence over time may be so dramatic that there is little doubt that they are real. The annual epidemics of measles in poorly immunized populations are usually reflected by even the worst surveillance systems. Less dramatic changes, however, may be the result of changes in the reporting system. An in-service training course or a new enthusiastic health worker in an area can produce apparent epidemics of disease through improved diagnosis and reporting. In the smallpox eradication programme the introduction of a surveillance system to identify new cases inevitably led to a large increase in the numbers reported. Conversely, numbers of reported cases may decline through loss of interest rather than the effects of a control strategy.

Place

Variations in incidence of disease by geographical area as recorded by routine health statistics are subject to misinterpretation if the coverage of service is not taken into account.

Aspects of coverage

Coverage may be defined as the percentage of people within a population who need and receive a particular service out of all those who need that service. This is usually measured at one point in time. Examples of coverage figures would be the percentage of leprosy patients in the population currently receiving treatment; the percentage of pregnant women making the requisite number of antenatal attendances; or the percentage of children under 5 who are fully immunized.

Data on the numbers of people receiving a service, i.e. *utilization*, depend mainly on analysis of existing records in clinics and hospitals. As described on page 153 the quality of records must be assessed before any analysis is carried out. Thereafter the daily number of attendances in each diagnostic category may be counted, or counts may be restricted to selected diseases. Diseases of local importance, such as diarrhoea, gonorrhoea, measles, or pneumonia, may be recorded in more detail, showing age, sex and address.

A service is utilized when patients perceive that they need it and then *demand* it. However, utilization may also reflect demand in the absence of need, for example people sometimes wish to have an X-ray because they believe it confers therapeutic benefit.

An analysis of coverage may be extended to include preventive and health promotion services. For example, what proportion of people use a clean water supply, have sanitation, attend health education meetings — if such exist? What proportion have access to newspapers or radios through which health education is or could be disseminated?

When analysis of coverage reveals a percentage that is markedly less than 100, as it usually is, it is necessary to determine the reasons. *Accessibility* of the service is a key factor and has three aspect — physical, economic and social.

Physical accessibility is the time required to travel to a service, e.g. a clinic. Obviously it depends on its topographical situation (e.g. on a hilltop or in the plains), and its position within the network of roads or other lines of communication. Its situation relative to the distribution and density of the population is also important. Work in Africa has suggested that a 10-mile radius from a hospital covers the distance which people will usually walk; a 20-mile radius takes account of public and private transport and the walking distance of nomadic peoples; a 30-mile radius defines the maximum area from which people will come except under special circumstances.

Physical accessibility may be expressed numerically in a variety of ways, according to the particular service and local circumstances. For example, the area within 1 hour's travelling time from a clinic may be mapped out, and the proportion of people living within this area out of all those notionally served by the clinic can be calculated. This calculation can be made using different travelling times for different services, e.g. antenatal or emergency. In choosing sites for a new service such as a mobile clinic it may be necessary to specify a minimum target, for example that every child should have a physically accessible service once a month.

Geographic variation of a disease may be explained in terms of demographic differences in the population. Age structure differences have already been discussed under standardization but variations in ethnic composition may also need to be adjusted for. The Fulani of The Gambia have a high prevalence of splenomegaly. Some groups of villages have high splenomegaly rates simply because they have a higher proportion of Fulani inhabitants.

Person

Socioeconomic influences may produce apparent differences in rates of disease.

Where people have to pay for health care, services may become economically inaccessible to the poor. An indication of whether this is occurring may be obtained by questioning users of the service about their occupational and economic circumstances. It may, however, prove difficult to obtain reliable information about the payments actually being made for a service, or to quantify poverty within the community.

A service may be both physically and economically accessible but yet have poor coverage because of social inaccessibility. The reasons why certain social groups do not use a service may be obvious, e.g. a language barrier, or they may originate in religious beliefs, taboos or fears. Older people may prefer traditional remedies; women may be shy of speaking about their medical problems; a new modern hospital may appear frightening.

Reasons for the lack of coverage of a service may be readily apparent to the outside observer, for example obvious causes of physical inaccessibility, or may become apparent as a result of informal conversations with local people, community leaders or traditional healers. Sometimes it may be helpful to carry out a questionnaire survey on a sample of the population not receiving adequate coverage. People are asked about illnesses they have had in the previous month, what medicines they have bought, consultations with traditional healers, use of any part of the health services, diseases they know to be common in the area (e.g. fever, haematuria, itching skin), and diseases for which they think suitable treatment is not available from the health services. This type of survey may also highlight high-risk groups for disease who are not currently being helped by the health service.

Cost-effectiveness

The design of an effective health service will require a balance in the use of available resources. Epidemiology will measure the effects of the services but these need to be related to other aspects of resources. Clearly the limiting resources of a health service are both financial and the availability of skilled personnel. An important aspect of the evaluation of the resources of a health service is the proportion of total resources given to primary health care.

Measures of this include the ratio of health service personnel in hospitals to those engaged in primary health care, the ratio of doctors to nurses and auxiliaries, and the recurrent costs of hospital services as a percentage of total recurrent costs.

It may be necessary to make periodic appraisals of the adequacy of supplies. During visits to clinics and other health facilities — visits which are best made without prior warning and at irregular intervals — a note may be made of such things as the availability of basic drugs, whether vaccines are being correctly refrigerated, and whether vehicles are being adequately maintained.

Efficiency

The resources needed for therapeutic and preventive services will depend not only on the actual medical procedures being carried out but on the way in which the services are organized and run. An assessment of the efficiency of a service will encompass a wide range of questions. Is the time of the health workers being used efficiently? Are they adequately trained and supervised? Are the various facets of the service properly integrated? Are the services directed towards the most prevalent diseases? Are expensive drugs being used when cheaper, equally effective ones are available?

Because health services everywhere are constrained by limited resources there is in consequence a pressing need to optimise the use of personnel and materials and thereby increase efficiency.

Outcome

If the achievements of health services are to be evaluated it is necessary for objectives to be agreed upon and defined. Thereafter the extent to which they have been fulfilled may be measured. Obviously evaluation will have to be restricted to a few selected outcomes, and the ease with which measurements are obtained will vary with the disease. For example, an outcome of an effective antenatal service, in which pregnant women are immunized against tetanus, will be the swift decline of hospital admissions for neonatal tetanus. In contrast the effectiveness of improvements in environmental sanitation in reducing the incidence of gastrointestinal disease will be more difficult to document.

Mortality data for the population will be of value but usually data on morbidity are required. As has been outlined earlier in this chapter, direct measures of morbidity or general indicators of the health and nutritional status of a community may be available from hospital and clinic records. When this is not so special surveys will be needed. The principles of these have already been outlined by reference to nutritional and leprosy surveys, where it was stated that the 'action' at the end of each survey included continuing evaluation of the nutritional or leprosy programme undertaken.

EPIDEMIOLOGY IN DEVELOPING COUNTRIES

This chapter has outlined some of the situations in which epidemiological techniques may be applied in developing countries. Application of these techniques will be fruitful in many aspects of medical endeavour: in the development of appropriate and effective health services, in the control of disease, and in the understanding of disease aetiology and natural history.

SUGGESTED FURTHER READING

Epidemiology

Benenson A S 1970 Control of communicable diseases in man. American Public Health Association, New York

Buck C, Llopis A, Najera E, Terris M 1988 The challenge of epidemiology issues and selected readings. Pan American Health Organization, Washington

Essex B J 1980 Diagnostic pathways in clinical medicine, 2nd edn. Churchill Livingstone, Edinburgh

Hutt M S R, Burkitt D P 1986 The geography of non-infectious disease. Oxford University Press, Oxford

Jellife D B 1966 The assessment of the nutritional status of the community. World Health Organization, Geneva

Kelsey J L, Thompson W D, Evans A S 1986 Methods in observational epidemiology. Oxford University Press, Oxford

Last J M 1988 A dictionary of epidemiology, 2nd edn. Oxford University Press, Oxford

Lucas A O, Gilles H M 1973 A short textbook of preventive medicine for the tropics. English Universities Press, London

MacMahon B, Pugh T F 1970 Epidemiology: principles and methods. Little, Brown, Boston

Robinson D 1985 Epidemiology and the community control of disease in warm climate countries. Churchill Livingstone, Edinburgh

Schelesselman J J 1982 Case control studies. Design, conduct analysis. Oxford University Press, Oxford

Statistics

Epidemiology and statistics methodology unit, WHO 1986 Sample size estimation: a user's manual. World Health Organization, Geneva

Health statistical methodology unit, WHO 1988 Adequacy of sample size. World Health Organization, Geneva

Kirkwood B R 1988 Essentials of medical statistics. Blackwell Scientific
  Publications, Oxford
Lindley D V, Scott W F 1984 Cambridge elementary statistical tables.
  Cambridge University Press, Cambridge
Swinscow R D V 1980 Statistics at square one, 6th edn. British Medical Journal,
  London

Social surveys

Abramson J H 1979 Survey methods in community medicine, 2nd edn. Churchill
  Livingstone, Edinburgh

Index